STILL STANDING

WHAT DOCTOR'S AND PHARMACEUTICAL COMPANIES
CHOOSE TO IGNORE

ILLINA LEFF

Illina Leff

ISBN: 0692988475
ISBN-13: 978-0692988473

STILL STANDING

DEDICATION

I would like to dedicate my book to my husband Bob and my kids
Noah, Joshua, Ryann and Nate for all the unconditional love and support
and giving me the Hope to always fight. I especially want to dedicate my
book to my girlfriends and the friends and family who have given me the
strength to get thru some of my hardest days. To my nieces and nephews,
I love and miss you. Special thank-you to my niece Seanna for helping me
with my book cover. To all those who suffer from Psoriasis and Psoriatic
Arthritis this book is for you. Keep fighting.

Finally, to my dear Mom and Dad, Thank-you for raising me to be the
strong woman I am today, I owe everything to the both of you.

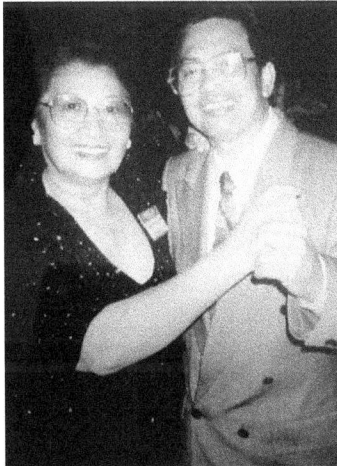

Illina Leff

TABLE OF CONTENTS

Illina Leff

ACKNOWLEDGMENTS

I would like to express my greatest appreciation to my doctors who have had to deal with one health issue of mine after another, I know I was not an easy patient. I would like to acknowledge my Doctors, Dr. Wetter and Interns and The Nurses at light therapy at Mayo Clinic Rochester who gave me hope and a reason to love ME again. A special Thank you to Charlie Goldsmith, The most amazing Energy Healer on earth. You have changed my life forever and I just love you! My therapist Carolyn, such an important person in getting me thru the hardest life moments. Last but not least, Thank -you Eli Lily for inviting me to share my story at your advisory board meeting. You gave me the confidence to share my story and validated that my story is worthy and I thank you.

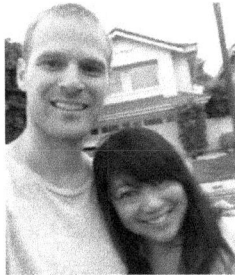

Thank-You Charlie Goldsmith

DISCLAIMER

This is a disclaimer that the truth and facts that are written and shared are solely from my experience and my journey. I am not stating that it has been proven that these drugs caused my side effect but I am sharing my coincidental experiences as stated on their products side effects. Some photos may be graphic.

Any medication that I have taken and may have suffered a side effect is what I experienced when taking the drug and by no means am I stating that it will happen to you or to not take the drug. We all take to medication differently, unfortunately I am that 2% who seems to be affected by side effects.

Medication is an important piece to healing and needed for quality of life and works better on some than others.

My goal is that doctors and pharmaceutical companies are aware of what patients will go thru when they put their trust in doctors and the drugs they prescribe.

I am not a professional writer and this book was written with a whole lot of love. As a first time author who will self publish my book, I hope to get my message across and beg forgiveness if not to your standards. Just trying to be true to myself.

1 "ALL YOU NEED IS ACUPUNCTURE AND A MASSAGE'

"Trust your gut instincts and never back down because it can be a matter of your life or your death." -me

"All you need is Acupuncture and a Massage." This would be the beginning of my experiences with doctors and lets just say "challenges"."

Some days I would just start to shiver and my face would become numb which also made me think that maybe I was having a stroke. I made an appointment with a doctor from a new group that was covered by my insurance. I remember meeting the doctor for the first time and he was young and very distant. Honestly, he acted like he was all that and a bag of chips! A bit arrogant that all I could think about was if I would be able to switch to a different doctor.

As a patient, I don't expect a hug or anything but I do believe a professional bedside manner is important. He made me feel like he had places to be and more important things on his mind and not focusing on his patient , ME at that moment.

After my exam he had mentioned that my blood pressure was really high and that it was probably stress and anxiety related.

I remember my days as slow and my mind was always in a fog. I was wondering if maybe I was suffering from postpartum depression since it had been about a year and a half since my daughter was born.

For the next couple weeks, I tried yoga and other exercises that would help relieve my stress, but with each passing day I felt worse and just could not function. I made a follow up appointment with my ever so caring doctor who told me that he would prescribe me Xanax and that would help me with my anxiety and depression.

I was in my mid 30's and I was definitely going thru a lot of stress. I was starting to think that maybe I did need to take Xanax. I found it really odd that he would not do any lab work on me. It felt like he already had a diagnosis from the beginning as a 30 something year old female, postpartum, suffering from anxiety and depression. But deep down I knew my body and these symptoms just did not jive.

I decided to change groups after months of not getting answers and the conclusion that I came up with was that I was just a female patient who kept pestering her doctors. I thought to myself "Maybe I needed to find a female doctor who would be more in tune with my symptoms."

It just happened that we were moving a couple towns over and I knew this would be a great reason to find a new female doctor who also practiced and encouraged Holistic Healing. I scheduled an appointment with my new female doctor and explained to her what I have been going thru. She seemed to understand what I was going thru and told me that male doctors sometimes do not understand female hormones and issues and that she would definitely be able to help me. I felt hope!

She did the basic lab work and the results showed it to be pretty normal with a slight elevation in my blood cell counts, and that I had nothing to worry about. Then it came… "All you need is Acupuncture and a Massage"

What? That's my diagnosis? That's the advice for why I have been feeling the way I have for months? I wasn't buying it but I guess I better schedule a massage and try acupuncture since of course it is what she ordered! My insurance does not cover acupunctures nor massages and it was draining my pocket along with the co-pays for my doctor visits. Did it help? It certainly felt good at the moment, but not really. I kept thinking to myself "What is going on with me?" Am I dying? Am I going to have a stroke or heart attack? This is NOT normal!

After going thru this for the past couple years now and my lady doctor was not pinpointing a solid diagnosis,
I decided that I would go and sit in my church which gave me a peaceful feeling and helped me to just cry it out. "What is happening to me? Please dear God give me the strength to overcome whatever it is I am going thru and help me get answers from my doctors, Please!"

I just need to get better and take care of my family.
Fast forward a couple months, I was still feeling weak and unable to function. I continued to suffer, but I was determined to find out what was wrong with me because whatever I was feeling, I knew was not right.

The answer to my prayers!!!!

It was time for my check up with my Obstetrician for my well check after having baby number four. So just to recap, I am going on almost 2 and a half years of trying to figure out what the heck was wrong with me. I love my doctor, Dr. Bailey, he has always been very thorough and so kind and always has the best bedside manners! After doing a thorough examination he says to me, "I feel a couple lumps on your neck, make sure you have your Internal medicine doctor check it out, it could be nothing, but just to be safe"

Once again, I made an appointment with my new lady doctor, you know the one who told me that all I needed was acupuncture and a massage, that one! I told her how my OB/GYN noticed a lump in my neck area and that he suggested to get it checked out. She then used the "Trust" card! She told me, "Fine, we will order a cat scan if you don't trust me!" I remember leaving thinking, did she just say that? Is it truly about not trusting you or the fear that another doctor was thorough in his examination and may have found something? To me, it was prayers answered, to her it was me doubting her, but as you will see, it made a difference in my life.

A few days later I received a call from her assistant, not the doctor, but her assistant saying to please come in and pick up my report. It showed that I had 6 nodules in my neck and she was NOW FINALLY referring me to an Endocrinologist so that they can be removed. My thoughts were wow, had my Ob/Gyn not felt my neck I would still be getting acupuncture and massages!

My new Endocrinologist did a biopsy and sent it away for expertise advice and according to their findings 3 doctors thought it to not be cancerous while 1 doctor said it would be and she told me that they had even made a bet to see who would be right.

Next thing I knew was that I was scheduled for surgery to have these nodules removed. I remember being really worried because months before, I had volunteered to help at my son's 8th grade dance and I was more worried about not being able to help out at his dance. With every surgery there is a risk, so I was scared "What if something happens?" The best thing I can do is say a prayer and leave it in Gods hands.

When I woke up from my surgery, I heard the nurses talking and all I heard was my name Illina Leff and the words "Total Thyroidectomy" at that moment I knew I had thyroid cancer since I was told before hand that if the biopsy comes back cancerous they will remove my thyroid.

Thyroid Gland:
The thyroid gland is a butterfly-shaped endocrine gland that is normally located in the lower front of the neck. The thyroid's job is to make thyroid hormones, which are secreted into the blood and then carried to every tissue in the body. Thyroid hormone will help the body use energy, stay warm and keep the brain, heart, muscles, and other organs working as they should

After having a Total Thyroidectomy, I was then scheduled to have radiation therapy for a week in what I called "THE DUNGEON" which was away in the basement of the hospital where everything was covered in plastic. The saddest thing ever was that if my family came to visit, they were only allowed to see me thru a small window the size of a mail slot. It was very hard and depressing, especially since I had my kids at home as young as a toddler.

So there you have it! After a few doctors later and a diagnosis of stress and anxiety and a prescription for Xanax and "All you need is Acupuncture and a massage" all I can say is I am so thankful to my Ob/Gyn the great Dr. Bailey, my angel for noticing the lumps in my neck after doing a thorough examination that my other doctors didn't do. This went on for two years of not feeling well. I was told the good news that the nodule was still encapsulated so it had not spread to my lymph nodes yet.

Definition:
Encapsulated: enclose in or as if in a capsule

I finally had the answer to why I was so tired, not being able to function, feeling cold and shivering which I told them from the beginning.

After this ordeal, I did feel that it was my job to let both doctors know that I was diagnosed with Thyroid Cancer. I felt that if I shared my experience, hopefully another patient will not go thru what I went thru. When I went to my lady doctor's office to talk to her, she would not come out. Her assistant told me that she was busy.
I really thought she was so unprofessional. She never went over my ultrasound results that showed my nodules, nor did she talk to mc after my surgery! Just her assistant. So odd.

Why did she not tell me my results? Was she upset or embarrassed? I just do not understand.

I was very happy to find a new internal medicine doctor who was very different and attentive and certainly not like my other doctors. I'm sure doctors do not want to be called out on their patient care and bedside manners, but come on, as a common courtesy, admit you made a mistake instead of having your assistant give you your results.
This is my life, and this could be yours and this is why I say "Trust your Instincts!

Seeing her pain and watching her struggle broke my heart often. She just has this warm heart and unstoppable attitude that was so contagious. I love her so much and am thankful the warrior that is inside of her.
-Kristy Banford

2 "YOU LOOK LIKE YOU ARE IN THE LAST STAGES AIDS"

"You look like you are in the last stages of Aids" is what my rheumatologist says to me. I can't say that I knew how to react to that statement. All I knew was that a couple of months ago he had prescribed to me a biologic that would help my Psoriatic Arthritis and my Psoriasis.
I remember being so confused trying to figure out if I had Psoriasis, Psoriatic arthritis AND Aids?

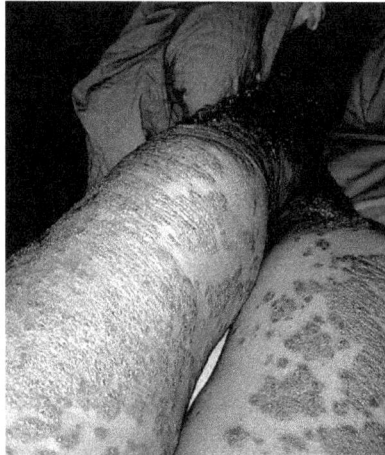

Why in the world would my doctor say this to me? Well, for starters my skin was covered in sores (See Picture) that looked like welts.

To my doctor it was Aids and not Psoriasis. My Rheumatologist suggested that I see a dermatologist so they can do further test.

However, he had a few questions for me. Questions that were very disturbing, questions that had me questioning my husband's fidelity. My doctor asked me how my relationship with my husband was and if I knew if he was being faithful. I had to take a moment to think about it, as far as I knew he was, but as I further analyzed what he was implying, it was that I may have contracted Aids from him!

So how do I handle this? How do I go home and tell my husband that they are going to test me for Aids?! How do I even look at my husband? All I knew was my doctor put the thought in my mind that my husband may be cheating on me and gave me Aids! What else can go wrong? Was this really happening?

I had an appointment with a dermatologist, she was petite, very soft spoken and very sweet. She looked me over and was very empathetic. She told me that they will take a sample of my sores and send it to the lab to get checked. They will do an Aids test, Herpes test, Gonorrhea and Syphilis test and suggested my husband do the same.

In the mean while, my doctor decided it would be best to take medication for Herpes to see if it will help clear the sores all over my body.

I remember leaving her office not knowing if I should cry or scream or beat my husband! But, I will keep my cool until the results come back. Now, I just had to play the waiting game and let my mind run wild with the worse possible scenarios. Why not add to the stress and go online and look at photos of AIDS patients and freak myself out even more!

The worse part was the waiting because honestly the picture was already painted thru my Rheumatologist questions. My husband was unfaithful, gave me Aids and I am going to die! I also had my skin for proof. I was sure I had Aids because he was a doctor, and he obviously knew from all his schooling, right?

I remember going to my church once again, no-one was there, it was very quiet and I asked God "What is going on?" Please give me the strength because I am scared of what might be. I felt like I was having Deja vu, back here at church saying a prayer. If I just put everything in your hands, it will happen the way it is meant to be and I believe everything will be okay. I need to remain positive.

 The days were going by slowly till my next appointment to get my results. In those days leading up to it, I found reasons to justify why my husband would have not been faithful. I felt like it was my fault. Who would want to be with someone whose skin was ugly from Psoriasis. I loved him but I also did not know if I should hate him. I just wanted to know the results. I was going crazy!

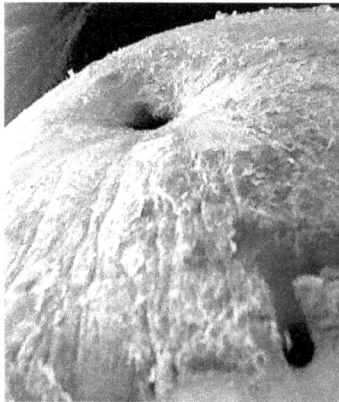

Finally, the day was here to get my results.
With Bob by my side, I knew that the news I was about to receive may end our marriage or we will breathe a big sigh of relief and there will be no other choice but to get stronger.

As my sweet doctor took out my chart, she looked at me and said "Your results are back and it looks like everything came back NEGATIVE, you do not have Aids, Herpes, Syphilis or Gonorrhea, but what you do have is in fact Psoriasis.

You are the 2% that got a side effect from the biologic that caused your Psoriasis to get worse.

My husbands comment "I knew it wasn't me."
But now what? I still look like I was in
the last stages of Aids and my skin was bleeding and in pain and my joints were killing me. I was told to stop taking my biologics and both my Dermatologist and Rheumatologist were going to work together to figure out what I could do.

My Thoughts:

What could my doctors have done differently:

I loved my doctor, Dr. Wherle, but he scared the heck out of me! My thought is that before you tell your patient they look like they are in the last stages of Aids, you should probably run all test to get accurate results. The fear is greater then the disease itself. The phrase "You look like you are in the last stages of Aids" was so scary and not only did it affect me mentally, it affected me emotionally. It had me think of every bad scenario possible! What did my doctor think would happen by saying this to me? Again, He was very kind, I really liked him but I think it sure could have been handled differently. I am hoping that what I write in my book would help a doctor think twice.

As for the pharmaceutical company who represented these biologics, I have been told that they noted my side effects and is now a clinical study. Though I did try to contact someone to share my thoughts on my side effects, no one has returned my call.

I have made it my mission to educate and share my story especially to the pharmaceutical reps who are at the booths every year at the arthritis walks.
When I approach the pharmaceutical booths to let hem know the side effects I have suffered from taking their drug, they either go silent, do not respond or they tell me that they have never heard that happen to anyone.

My Husbands Thoughts:

It felt like these Dr.'s couldn't figure out what was going on with her so instead of quietly running tests and going through the discovery process, they speculated and sent her deeper into depression and made her question my love for her. I can't believe their nerve and it pained me to keep giving them our business. I don't think most of them want to work hard to treat but instead they throw pills at her treating her like a lab rat. If these Dr.'s ran themselves thru clinical trials of the medication they prescribe, the landscape of the medical industry would look a whole lot different in a better way.

What amazes be about Illina is the mask she wears, even if she is in pain, shame or guilt she steps into daily life with a smile and compassion for others. -**Catherine Gadsby**

I think people are usually shocked when they find out or see photos of my Psoriasis because what you see in the photos above are covered when I am dressed up making me look "NORMAL". It's not like I go around flashing my skin. As for the Psoriatic Arthritis pain, I always get "You don't look sick". Unless I am in a wheelchair, you don't see arthritis pain. People go thru their days pretending their okay when we really are not. You just have to make the most of your days, make yourself feel the best you can and try to do it with a smile. Your family know how you truly feel. They don't have to hear it 24/7.

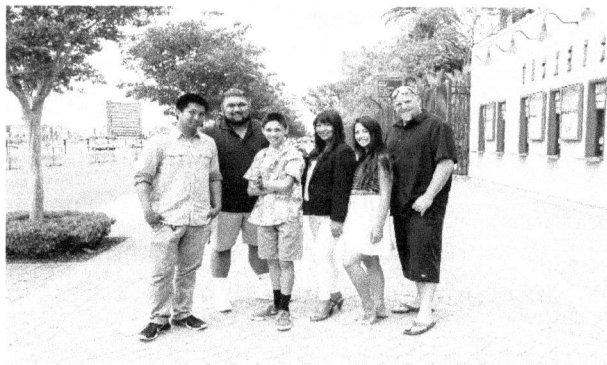

3 "YOU HAVE CANCER"

"Wait a second, where are we going? They are sending me
to an Oncologist again? Is this really happening? I just
went thru thyroid cancer and radiation a couple years ago! I
have cancer AGAIN? I thought I just had a bad cough or
Bronchitis? It's my daughter's birthday today… I just can't
think, hold on, my cancer is back, I'm going to die, I just
know it!"

My mind is racing and taking me to a bad place, AGAIN!
My anxiety level is causing my body to shake
uncontrollably. I am gasping for air because I cannot
breathe. My new family doctor has been treating me for my
Bronchitis, the diagnosis I was given with my prior medical
group. My other doctor was old, He seemed tired of his
job. He just kept giving me antibiotics and cough medicine.
But weeks were going by, and I was not getting better.
Taking a breath was a chore, but he told me that I just had
Bronchitis.

Blessing in Disguised

The new year was approaching to enroll for a new medical plan with my husband's work. After thoroughly looking at our options we decided a PPO would work best.
 But before I discovered I had cancer, I found this new medical group that I enrolled in.

I had a new doctor, he was very young, to me he was a Vietnamese Doogie Howser. He seemed really nice but sort of a Know it all. I told him about my Bronchitis and all the medications I was on, and next thing I knew he took out his handy dandy hand held medication dictionary of some sort.

Unlike my old doctor, he seemed very concerned and immediately ordered a chest x-ray. In my mind I was thinking how he wanted to see how bad my Bronchitis was. Hours later, I found myself back in his office and I could tell by his expression, I was about to be hit with news, and not good news. I want to tell you exactly what he said but after I heard "Your X-ray shows a huge mass in your lungs, I need you to see an oncologist ASAP" anything after that put my mind in a state of shock and once again the only thought was "I am dying!"

I heard the word Oncologist and I knew that only meant one thing and that was that I did NOT have Bronchitis and it could only mean that I had CANCER…AGAIN!

Dr. Pham, "How can this be?" He told me that one of the drugs that I was taking had a side effect that may cause me to have a cough and he needed to check it out.

I hurried to do my research on the current biologic I was on and how funny that the commercials that Phil Mickelson endorses have a disclaimer "May cause Lymphoma."

When I met with my new Oncologist, he seemed very short and to the point and was very attentive and concerned.

He looked at the X-ray that I had just taken and told me "You have a very large mass either in your lung or chest, we need to do a biopsy. The biopsy needs to be done so we know what kind of cancer you have and what treatment plan we need to put in place.

Huh? Excuse me? My fear went a next level up. My nerves were all over the place thinking how they were going to put a giant needle from either my back or side without puncturing my lung. All in the meanwhile I was wondering if being on this new and improved biologic would contribute to me having this mass in my chest. I had to try and put that out of my mind and get thru each of these test one day at a time. Instead of knowing I had Bronchitis which I thought would clear up with antibiotics and cough medicine, everything was different. I could not breath, I have cancer in my lungs or chest and I was so scared, I was wondering what I wanted to do incase this cancer kills me. My Bucket List!

After MRI's, Cat scans, X-rays and biopsies the result was in and my very smart gentle Oncologist says to me "You have Non-Hodgkin's Lymphoma. One of the largest masses I have seen and it is in your chest. We will need to start a very aggressive chemotherapy plan because surgery will not be an option.

Every appointment was worse then the other and I would just take a couple deep breaths. The worse part was sharing the news with my family. It was awful! I felt so much pain having to share this news. I hated it but after having a pity party, it was time to get things in order and fight. There was no other option, I had 4 kids and one was a toddler.

It was hard to tell the kids that I had Cancer again, but for us, it was best that we were truthful. We of course did not know what the plan was, or what God's plan was for me, but I just knew that we will be open and honest and live life and keep our household as normal as possible.

The one great thing about friends and neighbors was the overwhelming support that surrounded us. When you get news like this, you feel so lost but the kind gesture by friends and family was so powerful and greatly appreciated. I remember having a talk with one of my friends who brought up a great point. When someone you care for finds out they have cancer, sometimes you feel helpless and not sure how you can help and instead you stay away. That is the worse thing you can do especially if you are family.

I truly wished I had more of a support system from my family but for whatever reasons or excuses that I would come up with, it just did not make sense. The one thing that really hurt my heart was that I knew when you come from a Filipino family everyone would get together and do a prayer group, but for whatever reason, it never happened for me. I remembered how scared I was and I found myself going to my church.

I would sit there and pray and cry and pray when the church was empty. I would feel an overwhelming feeling of peace and I knew that I needed to stop worrying and to just put everything in God's hands.

I also remember kneeling with my eyes closed tears rolling down my face when a short old lady dressed in black with a black veil over her face came and touched me, and asked me what was wrong. She scared the heck out of me, I was thinking "Is this my angel of death coming to take me away?" She then laid on the floor and prayed so hard, also crying for my healing and I just had this feeling take over me and call me crazy but I knew that she was sent to me as an angel to help me thru this time. I just felt different and not so alone anymore. I had my eyes closed as she did this and when I went to thank her, she was gone. It was the weirdest thing. Was she real? I know she was!

As I went for my first chemo treatment, the nurses tried to gently stick me for my I.V. more then a few times. As if I was not nervous enough, I started to get a reaction to my I.V.

My face started to have a rash and then it traveled down my neck and my throat started to constrict.
I tried to wave at the nurses to get their attention but the room was full with other patients getting their chemo treatments as well.

I found myself looking around this room with about 25 other chairs and everyone was hooked up and I could feel the stares. They knew I was a newbie, and as I sat there for my six hour treatment, I can hear each of their stories.

They were young and old and some had the same cancer as I did and some looked strong and some did not.
I ended making a friend but I went home feeling really sad. She was a young mom with a brain tumor who had three young kids. She had been fighting this fight for awhile now and she said things did not look good. Hearing her story made me want to fast forward my life.

They would ask what my story was and I had to stop and think. When I explained my story I would tell them that I thought I just had Bronchitis but I have Non-Hodgkin's Lymphoma in my chest, but I started a new drug for my arthritis and all of a sudden I developed a cough. They would ask me if I got a side effect from taking the drug.

Everything had been a whirlwind and I never thought about it until till I had 6 hours of chemo to think about it. Did I get Lymphoma from this biologic? The first biologic I took coincidentally made my skin worse. Remember, I looked like I was in the last stages of aids but sure enough, the side effect said that 2% of patients with psoriasis will gets worse with the drug and that was me! I had six hours to do some research during my chemo treatments and I read the warning label which said "may cause Lymphoma or death or other side effects." Oh my gosh, am I going to lose my life because I tried this new drug to help the pain from my arthritis and my Psoriasis? My mind was spinning and I called my Rheumatologist right away to remind him about the first Biologic and Aids and now this! They were quick to call the Pharmaceutical company to let them know and my doctor informed me that every person has cancer that is dormant in them.

It just happened that with my immune system it was no longer dormant coincidentally after taking this new drug. Now I was angry and all I could think about was that everyone was full of it!

I really could not worry about that right now and I just had to put it aside to deal with later. I had a fight the fight and this chemo cocktail was making me feel horrible and made my hair come out in chunks. It started to itch and it was so uncomfortable. It was a bit strange but I found myself excited to lose my hair and get new wigs, long and short. I could not wait for Dr. Fong to give me a prescription so I can rush to pick up my new wigs. I knew losing my hair would be shocking for my family and I wanted to make light of the situation and try not to freak out the kids with a bald head so I had them each take a turn with the scissors and snip my long hair off. Afterwards, I looked in the mirror and my hair looked so stylish and cute, longer in the front and short in the back from my crooked hair cut but it was so darn cute.

However, I still had to find someone who would shave my head because it just kept coming out in chunks and I started to have patches all thru out my scalp. I had no idea what an ordeal it would be to have someone do this for me. I did not want my husband to shave my head because even though I knew he would, I felt that would shock him too. I went to a hair salon to see if they can shave my hair and the stylist was having a hard time so she styled my hair and could not stop crying. I didn't have the heart to keep traumatizing her so I left. A few days later I took my son to get his hair cut at our local barber shop when there was an Asian lady barber who was bald herself I was pretty excited and I knew she would shave my head!

I mentioned Asian because the reason for her bald head was not because she had cancer but because she just came back from a monk retreat of some sort. It didn't matter, she had no problem shaving my head and it felt so good! Chemo Cocktails are pretty powerful to make hair fall off!

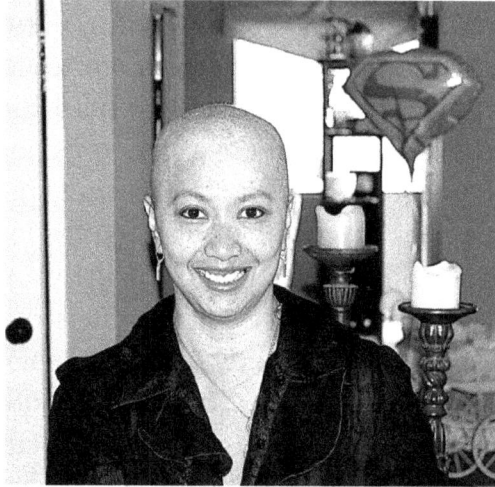

-As hard as we try none of us will ever understand the daily struggles she goes through just to make it to tomorrow
-Amy Kiikka Lalonde

I felt this was part of cancer and even though it was an easy process for me, I realized when I went to the wig store how devastating it was for other woman to lose their beautiful locks of hair and trust me, I get it! For some of us, our hair is our Superman Cape or our security blanket. If we can just remember it will grow back and concentrate on fighting the fight. Let's just wear cute wigs get dolled up and live life. Now years later, some of my friends who talk about when they met met me back then would say they had no idea what I was going thru because I acted like I was "Normal" when really, I was giving my all to pretend I was ok when I really was not.

My Thoughts:

When you get diagnosed with the "C" word, you automatically wonder "Am I going to Die?" and you can't help but freak out. But then you also start to see things in a whole new light. The tree that you use to drive by a million times and never noticed becomes a beautiful tree of life so vibrant and alive! The clouds are beautiful and blue and each day with family is more precious then the next.

I just could not understand my life, I just had thyroid cancer and now Non-Hodgkin's Lymphoma and I thought to myself, God is telling me something here and giving me a chance in life so I better live it! It would be nice if the pharmaceutical company of the drugs I took would acknowledge me and return my calls.

4 "YOU ARE A POSTER CHILD FOR SIDE EEFECTS"

Being told that I was the Poster Child for side effects was not exactly how I wanted to be labeled. When my sweet dermatologist said that to me, I was thinking "Goodness, that is really sad." But honestly, that pretty much summed me up to a tee.

When this all started I had an HMO and I was assigned to their doctors. Once their doctor saw you and thinks you need a specialist, you have to wait for an approval and sometimes that can take forever! I remember one day I had an appointment with my Oncologist which now a days your doctors are able to pull you up in their system to check your history, your lab work and any other test that has been done within the group and what medications have been prescribed to you. On this particular day however, they had my physical chart, which when I saw it was two charts as thick as the big yellow page book from the olden days if anyone remembers those.

Even my new Oncologist Dr. Fong was like "Wow! this is thick!" I think the reason he had my physical chart was to go thru my health history of good, bad and ugly!

I honestly get so overwhelmed with all my different doctors that it gave me anxiety to the point of a melt down. Since I had so many issues, the normal protocol was that you see your main Internal Medicine doctor, and since I have a PPO insurance my cop-pay for that doctor is $30 a visit. Once he figures out what is wrong, he then refers you to a specialty doctor which then becomes $45 a visit. For me it was a Rheumatologist for my joints to diagnose my Psoriatic Arthritis, a Dermatologist for my skin who treated my Psoriasis, A Cardiologist for my heart, who treated my heart failure and an Endocrinologist for my Thyroid Cancer and Diabetes. Also my Ob/Gyn for woman health issues and last but not least, my Oncologist who was treating my Non-Hodgkin's Lymphoma.

It was like a puzzle trying to figure out what was wrong and I was so overwhelmed with one appointment after another. The co-pays were outrageous along with the drive and the parking fees. This was like a full time job and whatever they were saying to me was going in one ear and out the other because I was so overwhelmed! I could not keep track and I began to wonder, how do elderly people with health issues keep track of appointments and medication? I finally told my main doctor that we had to come up with a plan. I could not do this any longer and he needed to stop sending me all over the place. He actually understood and decided to call them and explain what was going on and that he would handle my other issues for now I felt that getting admitted to the hospital was so much easier.
My doctors all came to me and the lovely nurses prepared my medication and the food nutrition would serve me a nutritious, low calorie, low salt diet. It made being sick a piece of cake.

I know that I shared a laugh with my Dermatologist when she told me that I was the poster child for side effects but then what? Will I ever get better? My Rheumatologist put me on biologics and I was suppose to trust him that this drug would help, but instead my Psoriasis got worse and all of a sudden I am taking an Aids test? Even my Oncologist would do chemo treatments and I remembered how I would have a reaction to the chemo which cause the side of my face to swell and turn red leaving me unable to swallow.

Getting these side effects are a scary thing and even though you do not want to take these medications that are suppose to help you, it takes over your mind and you start to think, what happens if I get this or that and what is worse is when you actually suffer a side effect. Once that happens you don't even want to try anything else, especially if it is new.

Even though they have clinical trials or they ask you to be in a clinical trial, I do not want to be the tester to see what can go wrong. There are so many new drugs out there that offer to help you if you join their clinical trial, but for some reason I can never qualify since I have had cancer. Maybe it will affect the trial if you get cancer when taking their drug.

Then you get the people who ask you "Why even take the drug?" It gets to that point when you haven no quality of life and you are weak and in a wheelchair that you have weighed your options and say "Do I take the risk of taking the drug and something might happen, or do I just lay here everyday in pain suffering and just wither away and die?" When you are desperate, you will do and take anything! Its part of the fight and the Will to live. Honestly, it can't get any worse.

So what qualified me to be the poster child for side effects? I took a Biologic and I was told that I was that 2% that my Psoriasis got worse and that is when my doctor told me I was in the last stages of Aids. I can't make this up. It is on

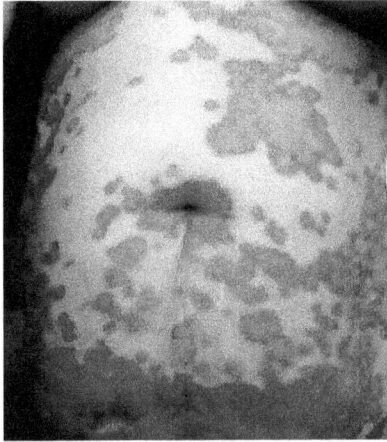

their warning label. The second biologic I took I coincidentally got Non-Hodgkin's Lymphoma and I would always see this on their commercials and of course on their warning labels. I decided to try a third biologic and coincidentally, once again, I ended having heart failure twice! I think that is how I would be deemed "The Poster Child for Side Effects"

I am not exactly sure why this was happening to me, but it does not mean this drug will cause the same side effect in someone else. I have stated this in my other chapters that my story is not your story, nor will it be yours. The best thing is to try different things and just hope it goes well. If not, just pay attention to your body and keep your body in check. It is perfectly ok to know and research the drugs that are being prescribed and ask your doctors questions, state your fears and concerns.

Most drugs that you take, you can usually stop and get it out of your system. When you have a good team of doctors looking out for you, they will work together and get you back on track.

I knew that drugs were not my friend, but I also knew that there are so many new drugs that will be available and I am confident I will find something safe one day. In the mean time, I also try healthy, natural alternatives to treat my Psoriasis. I decided to go to the Mayo Clinic in Rochester Minnesota to seek out the Goeckerman Treatment which I know I have mentioned in another chapter. This treatment consisted of Tar and light therapy and it was a natural alternative. It was a long treatment of having to be in the Mayo Clinic for a month, but I felt confident that this would work for me, and it did wonders for me.

I live in California, and it sure was not close, but if I had my choice, I would fly there every year and stay there for one month to get the treatment. The Doctors, interns, nurses in the light therapy room were so amazing. I left there with a great experience and a new group of friends

My Thoughts:

It is hard especially when you experience side effects to continue trying new things but it's ok to have an open mind and try what maybe out there in the universe to try. I had the opportunity to meet and Energy Healer, Charlie

Goldsmith who opened my eyes to something new and exciting. Yes, people might be skeptics but hey, what have you got to lose!

He certainly helped me with my arthritis and at this moment while writing this book, I feel great! I need to stop waiting for the day when whatever he did will go away and just embrace every day. I will keep searching for healthy alternatives because I need to know just incase my kids ever have to deal with Psoriasis or Psoriatic Arthritis that I have researched safe and healthy alternatives.

"I've watched you suffer and struggle for years, wondering what I could do to help when you have tried so much only to not get better or sometimes get worse.
                                        -**Kira Olander**

My Ugly Truth
Psoriasis and Psoriatic Arthritis

Do I have to get up today?
I feel like I just laid my head on my pillow,
Am I able to get up today?
My body just won't let me

Does anyone even know, Can you see it in my eyes
I know I am silent but I am screaming inside!

I am disgusted with myself, I cannot even look in the mirror
Wow, is that really me? How ugly, How ugly, How ugly!!!

What are these sores, these scales that cover me? What are these flakes that
fall and fill my bed? They hurt and sometimes bleed, I cannot help but try to
scratch them off, and this is why I cannot sleep, I feel my skin burn as my tears start to
fall, this cannot be me, not beautiful at all ....

I miss my soft skin, I missed being caressed, your eyes notice others but I understand, I
would feel the same, I feel the disgust, I am so so sorry, you don't deserve this ugly me

If that were not bad enough, my body struggles to stand and take a step
Why are my fingers black and blue, why can't I do something as easy as get myself
dressed? My hands are not my friend, Why me, why me???!!!!

Psoriasis you make me feel so ugly! Psoriatic Arthritis you bring me so much pain! But
you will not define me! I HAVE to get up and face the truth! I will fight you every minute
of every day because there is no other option than to fight... I will fight thru this pain and
thru these tears.

As much as my body is tired, as much as I want to crawl back into bed, its just not
going to be my ugly truth because you just don't define me.

5 "DO YOU HAVE A WILL OR ADVANCE DIRECTIVE"

As the team of nurses, technicians, therapist and E.R doctor were quickly hooking me up to various tubes to monitor my heart and blood pressure, I could sense that there was something really wrong happening to me, once again! Here I am again, it's a pattern now, and I am wondering if this is it this time? My heart is racing and all I could think about are my kids since my husband was already right beside me.

Let's go back a couple weeks. I recall that I was not feeling well and every time I would walk short distances I was so winded. I have never felt this way and this was something new. Once again I found myself trying to figure out what was going on. What have I been doing differently? Have I taken any new medication that might cause me to feel like this? Do I have the flu or a virus of some sort? Why yes, just a couple months ago I was at my worse again, a flare up, my autoimmune disease was taking its toll on my body. I was pretty bad.

When will this end? Not sure how many more times I can go thru this.

It had been a few years since being on Humira and Enbrel and possible coincidences with the side effects from these biologics. I am fearful of going back to my doctors because I know that they will just prescribe another drug.
In fact, last time I had an appointment with my Rheumatologist, I can see he was getting a bit frustrated. I just went thru months of chemo for my Non-Hodgkin's lymphoma for goodness sakes. You bet I was scared of trying another drug. I am not sure why my doctor cannot understand the reasons why I was so scared.

What makes me give into another drug? Having a severe form of Psoriasis and Psoriatic Arthritis. Being told I am top 10% worse in the nation. Plain and simple, the pain and the suffering. For some it maybe mild, but for me it hits me hard like a ton of bricks. I tend to get very weak, unable to walk from the Psoriatic Arthritis that I am once again using a wheelchair and a walker and the pain is so unbearable, worse then giving birth! My Psoriasis also takes over my body, itchy red patches, skin all over the place. Sometimes I can fill half a cup with dry skin in a day, not to mention how my skin will bleed from scratching it raw. When I pass by a mirror I cannot even bare to look at myself. And yes, that would be after taking this ointment, this cream a soothing bath, changing my diet, you name it. The depression sets in, I cry after everyone leaves the house and scream "Why me?!!!" How did I get this lottery of arthritis called Psoriatic Arthritis and skin problems called Psoriasis? It is bad enough having one, but to have both! Yup, I hit the lottery!

I'm embarrassed and disgusted, I just want to curl up in a corner and never leave my room. But then I have to shake it off and remember that it's ok to have a brief pity party and then remember, I have kids to take care of.

I need to show them that I will fight and never give up. Which takes me back to why I keep trying a new drug at any cost.
I am slowly dying and my quality of life is non existent. I am hopeful that there has to be one drug out there that will work for me!

I was introduced to ANOTHER Biologic. It was another injection and it wasn't quite the same as the previous biologics that I took so I was up for the challenge. I agreed with my sweet dermatologist that it was about my quality of life and if I didn't do anything, I would just suffer from my disease.

I decided to take it and pretty much in a week things were looking up for me. My skin cleared up and I was able to walk pain free. My joints were not cracking and I was hopeful but scared. It is always in the back of my mind wondering what will be my next side effect.

A month into taking this, I started to put two and two together again. Could this be why I am so winded and cannot even walk from my bedroom to my kitchen? I remember attempting to go to Disneyland with the kids and did not quite make it half way to the entrance and we had to go home.

My anxiety was starting to take over me and I felt like passing out. I decided to wait till the next morning to see my Internal Medicine doctor and once at his office he set up an appointment with a cardiologist but not after telling me that he thought I maybe about to have a heart attack and to go to the emergency room immediately! WHAT??? Are you kidding me?

So this is what brings us back to the beginning. I was in the emergency room while all the nurses and techs tried to get my blood pressure under control I think it was over 220/120 and they were frantically hooking me up to tubes and brought in the crash cart and that is when the E.R. doctor came in and asked me the magic question "Do you have a Will or an Advance Directive?" If something were to happen to me like death or if I became unresponsive, who would be in charge to make decisions? Bob my husband was sitting next to me, not sure what was going thru his mind, but I turned to the doctor and was like "Why? am I dying?" She told me that I maybe about to have a heart attack and the reason I have been feeling the way I do is because I was going into heart failure.

My life all of a sudden just flashed before my eyes. Every birth, every birthday, my wedding, every milestone was whizzing thru my mind as the E.R. team was hooking me up to every tube and rolling in the crash carts. All I knew, was that I wanted to see my kids before this heart attack was going to take place. Then to answer the doctors question, I am in my mid 40's, never thought of having a Will or Advance Directive, which I probably should have thought about when I was going thru my cancer.

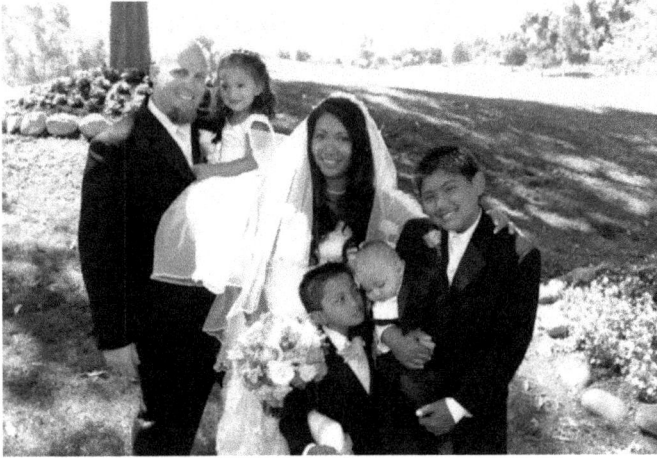

Oh my gosh, am I never going to see my family again?
What a coincidence AGAIN, to know that this heart failure
maybe due to a side effect of the latest drug I had taken.

How can I be in heart failure? How can it not be a side
effect? I don't think I will ever find out if I have a heart
attack and die! Like all the other drugs, whose to say that
this is a side effect indicated on their product. You just
can't pinpoint it, but it sure seems coincidental that I end
up getting "similar" side effects after taking certain drugs.
Honestly, this episode shocked me and I was not prepared.
Think about it. If you are asked that question laying in the
emergency room "Do you have a Will or Advanced
Directive?" What would go thru your mind? That was the
worse feeling ever.

I did not end up having a heart attack thanks to the E.R team getting everything under control but I still had to go thru quite a few test with my new Cardiologist to find out why I was going into heart failure. I did end up getting admitted into the hospital after this whole ordeal. I was told that the next thing would be to check and see if I had a blockage in my heart and if surgery would be the next step. It was very comforting to hear from different nurses daily how my Cardiologist really knew his stuff and everyone raved about him. It is always reassuring to hear things like that. On a side note, I also want to give kudos to all the nurses out there. I have been pretty lucky with getting some awesome nurses while in the hospital.

I noticed that being a nurse really takes a certain person to take on such a job. Nurses to me are like Angels!

My doctor finally had results and surprisingly he said there was no blockage in my heart area and no surgery was needed. That was good to know, but why did I have this near death experience? He even asked me if I had been experiencing a great amount of stress which could have put my heart in shock.

He also told me to get off the biologic that I was on since that was the newest thing I was on. I was put on a couple of new meds to treat my heart failure and taught a new saltless diet. This whole thing was just strange to me. One moment I am at deaths doors and then the next I am fine! Once again, they do not address the possibility of a side effect but that it may possibly be stressed related.

My Thoughts:

It was really scary to hear the words "Do you have a Will or an Advance Directive?" My life did flash right before my eyes! All I kept wondering was will I see my kids again? After all the testing and no solid indication for my heart failure, how could I not think it was another reaction to the latest medication. I'm not trying to knock these drugs or pharmaceutical companies but it is certainly a coincidence and it is my reality. I want to point out that what happens to me does not mean it will happen to you, nor am I saying do not take these drugs. We take it to find THE magic drug that will bring us relief and to give us our life back.
As for having a Will or Advance Directive, you are never to young, it's definitely the best idea, most especially for a person like me with so many health issues.

My Husbands Thoughts:

My heart dropped and my life flashed before my eyes. Once I came back to, I realized how un-prepared we were. I thought there was no way we were at the point in our lives we needed or I even thought about having one of these. We are still young enough that neither of us thought we would need this at this point in our lives.

Will

A will is a legal document that tells what a person wants to have done with their property after their death.

Advance Directive

It is a legal document that should be signed by a competent person to provide guidance for medical and health-care decisions like when a person may be on life support in the event the person is unable to make decisions.

" Through all her difficult obstacles, this super woman manages to place everyone's needs before hers! "
-QUIN HYLAND

6 GOODBYE LETTERS

Who would ever think that there would be a day that I would be writing good-bye letters to each one of my kids? Well that day came for me and I am sure that this has happened to other parents out there who have been faced with a life threatening illness. No, it was not because I was suffering from an autoimmune disease, but it was because I was diagnosed with Non-Hodgkin's Lymphoma. As you read in my previous chapter "You Have Cancer" this was a very difficult time in my journey of journeys!

I was having a hard time breathing, gasping for air and not sure if I was going to wake up each morning. They first thought I had was that I had Lung cancer but it ended up being a huge mass in my chest that was inoperable and I was diagnosed as having Non-Hodgkin's Lymphoma. Chemotherapy treatment would have to work to put me in remission.

I already put it in my mind that I was going to fight as hard as I could not just for my life but for my family. They need me, but in the back of my mind, what if? What if I don't make it? After all, I sat in a room full of other patients who were all there for chemo and some who had the same thing I did. The reality was that I made friends and got to know their stories. One day they would be there, and another day I would never see them again.

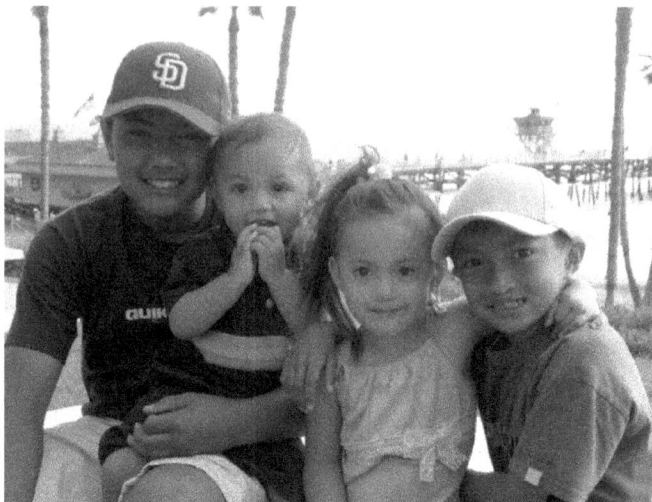

I would not see my new friend again because they had passed away. That could be me. Who was to say that my chemo would not work for me. No one knows.
It didn't help when my doctor would tell me that this is the biggest mass he has seen in anyone's chest.

All I knew was that I will fight, but I also need to be prepared. I found myself pulling back from the kids a bit. I did not come home and cry and hug them tight as often as I could. I should have, I know they were scared. I had cancer, I lost all my hair, it is scary!

I felt that if I were to emotional it would worry them. I just wanted to keep busy and create memories and if I did not come out ahead in this fight, they would not be so broken.

At the time the kids were 3, 5, 9 and 13 years old. I started to make plans on how I needed to teach my kids some basic necessities just in case.

As their mom I usually did everything for them like cook, clean and do their laundry but I wanted to make sure that they learn how to do this for themselves. I started to teach them these simple life skills. Some of my friends thought it was funny how my kids would wash their own clothes and and put them away later on. I mean, I was not dropping them off at a laundry mat with loads of laundry or anything, it was a simple "Ok kids, follow me, we stick the clothes in the washer, put some soap and press START, we then put it in the dryer and take it out and put it away" For one thing, it helped me since I was weak and not able to handle my normal mom duties but I could also notice a sense of responsibility.

The next thing I would do is have them help me and teach them simple recipes so they would not starve. I did notice two out of the four really like to cook and the other two liked being served.

They also had house cleaning chores and taking care of our pets. It was important that I did not have a housecleaner come, though I needed one, but again it was important for me to teach my kids some important life skills. Some parents would rather not have their kids do these kind of things but it was important to me as a mom who may not survive her cancer to instill these valuable lessons. I wanted to make sure that when they are out in the real world, they will be able to survive.

Which now brings us to the letters. Just imagine writing a good bye letter to each one of your kids. Where do you begin and what exactly would you say?

I could not write just one letter to all four of them, they each have different personalities and their ages ranged from the age three to thirteen years old.

As I wrote each letter, each sentence was harder then the one before. My tears soaked the stationary. How was I going to get thru this? I had to and I did. I let each one of them know how proud I was of them. I highlighted their strengths and how they are the greatest gift given to me by God! I told them to reach for the stars and dream big and to treat others with respect and to be humble and kind.

I let them know that from the moment they were born how I was overwhelmed with joy and a love so great you cannot even explain it. Each and every milestone in their life will forever be in my heart and I can only share how it made me one very happy mama!

I went down memory lane with each of them and I cried uncontrollably just thinking of them having to read this. I did find peace being able to write this because how many parents can do this for their child if they died a tragic and sudden death? I actually found myself blessed.

Obviously, I am still here today to tell my story. These letters are tucked away in a box somewhere, they never had to read it because thankfully I beat cancers butt and I am in remission. The kids are now 13, 16, 20 and 23 and I could not be more proud to be able to watch them grow and become the best humans possible. I always say to myself, If I were to die tomorrow, I will die happy and I know my kids will be okay.

My Thoughts

Will my kids ever know that I took medication prescribed by my doctors that may have coincidentally caused me to suffer a side effect? Could these Biologics have been responsible for my Non-Hodgkin's Lymphoma or me looking like I was in the last stages of AIDS or having heart failure twice? Maybe not, but why does the commercial or the packaging say "May cause Lymphoma or sometimes death" A coincidence again I'm guessing. Do the pharmaceutical companies know what becomes of the patients that took their drug and all of a sudden has Lymphoma and is now writing Good-Bye letters to their children? The impact is so much more! Yes, it may help thousands of other patients and that makes me happy, but how about the silent side effect sufferers? This is what happens to the families. I'm not sure they truly know. I can't say that they are to concerned since no one returns my calls. It just seems that if I took a chance trying YOUR drug that just maybe you can take a second to listen to what I have experienced. Do I matter? For me, this is my journey and I just have to go with it. As far as writing Good-Bye letters to my kids, I don't think these doctors or pharmaceutical companies understand until they have walked in my shoes. No one should be writing good-bye letters to their kids! Write "I Love You letters" now while you are good and healthy! It is okay to let them know how proud you are of them or even things you wish for them. You just never know. Sometimes tragedy strikes and you never get that chance.

My letter today

Dear Family,

I love you so much! Thank you for being my family and for all the years you all have been by my side. Even at my worse moments, you loved me and did not judge me and were able to understand that I was not contagious and still hugged me.

I am so proud of the humans you have become and I so enjoy when we get together and create more memories.

Remember to always fight and never give up and to pray during the darkest moments in your lives which I hope will be very few or none at all. But most especially, be there for one another as brothers and sisters. The strongest love you can show is support in their time of need.

I Love you all Forever,
Mom

Through good days and bad, her perseverance and hope are gifts she shares with inspiring optimism.
  -Linda Howard

I asked my kids what memory or thought they may have of how it has been to have a sick mom, Here is what they wanted to share:

Noah 24 Years old

My mom had to face adversity and death when it was at her doorstep. She is the definition of having strength in the mental aspect and someone I look up to very much. In my freshman year of high school, she was diagnosed with Non-Hodgkin's Lymphoma cancer. Despite the grim news that she received, she looked at getting cancer a different way. A way that opened her eyes and appreciate life to its fullest. She is the strongest person I know mentally because of the way she took this situation. After numerous chemo and radiation treatments my mom fought through this life changing event. The support from family and friends our family received during this time gave her the strength to keep fighting and not give up on life.

Joshua 20 Years Old

When my mom was sick I don't think I understood how serious the whole situation was. I remember not having a lot of answers and feeling helpless as I saw my mom not being able to get up in the morning. Whenever my friends asked me why I was late or didn't even show up to school sometimes because my mom couldn't drive, I wouldn't know what to say. My parents would tell me not to worry and that they're handling it so I tried to think about other things. I would think about baseball or try to read but my mom would be in the back of my mind wondering if she's okay at that moment.
When I was at school and she wasn't doing too well that morning she would be in the back of my mind.

Ryann 15 Years Old

Most of the memories I have of my mom are from the time her sickness was debilitating her the most. I remember at just four years old hearing my mom scream and cry in pain and thinking to myself "what can I do to help her?" Making lunches for myself and my brothers were one of the few simple tasks I took on to help out around the house, while I also remember helping her put her clothes on, aiding her around the house, starting the car for her, and other simple activities most healthy people take for granted. I remember laying in her bed with her having talks about what we would do if she were to die right then and how she would show us how to take care of ourselves by teaching us simple cooking recipes, how to do our own laundry, etc. I remember as a little kindergartener and first grader seeing other kids' moms helping out in class and wondering "how come my mom doesn't do that?" As I got older, my weekdays consisted of getting to school late because my mom wasn't able to pull herself out of bed or not even getting to school at all because her body was in such agonizing pain. After school it was always straight to the doctor's office for checkups and sitting in the waiting room with my younger brother, wondering what news our mom had for us next. Those days, although bad, weren't the worst I remember, though. The days I remember the most are the hospital days. Normally my mom would pick my brother and I up from school, but the days when my dad or my moms friends would pick us up we're the days I knew something was seriously wrong.

We'd drive over to the hospital and I'd see my mom hooked up to all these machines and tubes, but she always put on a brave face for us. That's one of the things I Love most about my mom, she's so strong and always considers others before herself. We'd stay in her room with her all day and when it was time to go, I'd cry and not want to leave. We'd go home without her and I would always sleep in my dads bed with him because I was so scared for my mom and what the future would hold for our family.

Nate 13 Years old

As a young boy, my life was different then most of my friends. Most kids would have their moms make them breakfast and make them lunch, they would have their mom drive them to school everyday. But my mom taught me how to make my own breakfast, make my own lunch, get myself ready for school, because she was unable to do that for me. My life when she was sick was mostly helping my mom. Some days I had to help her start the car, and some days I had to help her put her clothes on and push her in the wheelchair. Most of my days were spent in the doctor's office with her or helping her with anything she needed. Some days, she wasn't able to take me to school, so I biked or skated their, and some days I had to miss school so I could push her in her wheel chair at her doctor's appointments.

It is definitely hard to know that these are the memories my kids have of me. I know coincidently having some of the side effects from the various drugs that were prescribed was not intentionally done by my doctors or pharmaceutical companies, but once I did suffer a side effect, it just seemed like what happened to me was not that important in their books. They have no idea what my family went thru. I don't have the solution to what should be done, but we are people who put trust in a drug you prescribed or you manufactured. Not only does it seem that when I called I was made to me feel like I am wasting their time and yes it does make one angry. I absolutely think there should be some kind of compensation for the pain and suffering for what a families go thru along with the financial burden that comes with hospitalization and treatments to now correct what has most likely been caused by a side effect from a drug that everyone tries to say "No, It's not from OUR drug" COINCIDENTALLY.

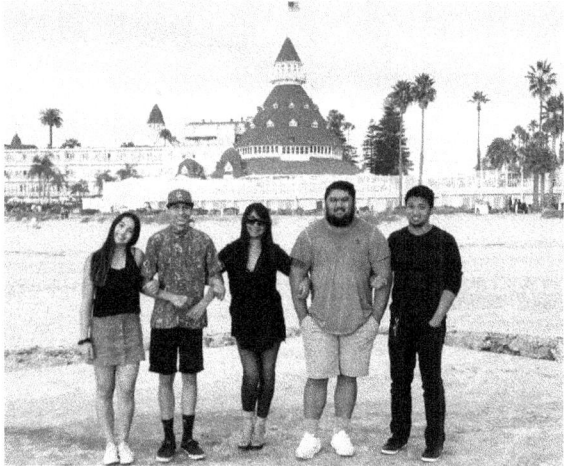

7 IT'S OKAY IF YOU WANT TO DIE MOMMY"

What would posses my daughter to tell me that it would be okay if I wanted to die? She must have been about nine or ten years old and I remember the exact moment when she said this to me.

Ryann was about three years old when I started to deal with all my medical issues. I believe she was my little angel sent to me to get thru all of the hardships that were about to

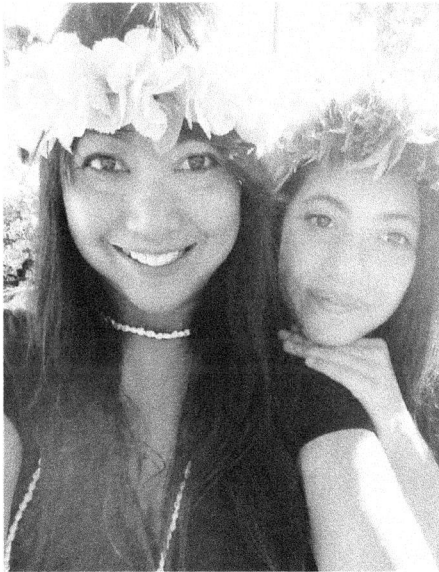

come my way. I have three other boys, two which were even older than her, but I can't even explain how at age four she was taking care of me and even her older brothers without being told. I would catch her going into her brother's room and making their bed or even folding laundry.

I was in the very beginning stage of my arthritis when I had no idea what I was dealing with. All I knew was that I could not even walk, start my car or get dressed. At four years old she would swoop right in and help get me dressed, and basically do everything for me.

This was a difficult time because I can see how scared the kids were wondering what was wrong with their mom.

I could not even explain it because I did not know myself. All I knew was that God had sent me my own angel to get thru these difficult days. I did have my husband Bob, but it was hard to turn to him and ask him to help me get dressed from head to toe. I was embarrassed and humiliated. All I could think about was "What is wrong with me? I am not the girl he married" and I could see the fear in his eyes. Every day I got worse, my body was in so much pain and doing something as easy as walking to the bathroom was no longer possible. He would have to carry me and gently place me on the toilet and come back to put me in bed.

It was great when he was here but what if he needed to go to work? I had to figure something out and I had him get me a walker that I would place next to my bed along with a bucket incase I could not make it to the bathroom. Yup, this was my life and I was very humiliated and the thought kept playing in my mind "Is this going to be me for the rest of my life?"

I could NOT bear the pain and I was just going thru such a depression and my kids could see my pain and suffering.

I tried to hide my pain and I tried not to cry but it was hard. I didn't want to scare my kids.

I did not want to be a Debbie Downer to my friends and family every time they called. I just felt so bad crying and being so depressed that I was starting to have bad thoughts of taking my life because I could not bear the pain. I just did not want to put my family thru this.

I reached out to family and shared what I was going thru, but I think I scared them because they just did not come around. I felt so abandoned. It would have been nice to have the support to help me with my kids at a time I could not.

So here I was, unable to walk, get myself dressed or take care of my family. I had sores all over my body and the pain was just to much to take. Even going to the doctor was such a big production and I now needed to add a wheelchair to the mix.

It would take me 30 minutes just to walk from my bedroom to the front door. This was my new ritual every day trying to take my kids to school, to the point where the school would call me to ask why the kids are always late and if there are arrangements that can be made to get them there on time. I felt like a horrible mom.

Since we had moved a few times, I didn't have a support system where I knew parents or felt comfortable asking for help. Again, my family was either way to far or I didn't want to burden them. I felt like they knew what I was going thru, and I would ask for help but it would become an ordeal.

I was getting more disappointed asking for help and hearing their excuses and I knew I was not about to beg. I knew that whatever was in store I needed to get it handled with my husband, my kids and whatever friends that were willing to help us out. I knew I was going to be okay.

When I was able to finally get the kids to school I would just cry and crawl back into bed trying to come up with a game plan of how I was going to pick the kids up from school. How am I going to go on living like this? I didn't want to live. This wasn't a quality of life!

At this moment I wasn't thinking about how my doctors can help me, I was thinking how I could not bear the pain and how awful I look and it started to consume my day. I was alone and all I kept thinking is how can I end this suffering? How? Should I take these sleeping pills? Should I crash my car into a pole? Should I take this plug from the vacuum cleaner and wrap it tightly around my neck?

This is how powerful this disease was! I was not able to eat because of the pain. I was not able to function as a mom or a wife because of the pain. Even laying in bed going onto one side to another was a challenge because of the pain. My legs felt like bricks and my blankets were covered in spots of blood from my skin cracking and bleeding. Who in their right mind wants to live a life like this. My doctors were even baffled and shocked since apparently I am the worse patient with this disease they have ever seen. Seriously? I was losing all hope.

Was I being selfish wanting to die? I am able to justify why I should take my life! My prayers were not "If I die before I wake" they were "Please dear God, just put me out of my misery and I don't want to wake up".

My Ryann could sense my pain, she out of everyone in the family saw my suffering and one day she laid next to me with her arms around me and said "It's ok if you want to die mommy".

What child would say that to her mommy? What child would have courage to say that? As I write this with tears streaming down my face, I remember the comfort she brought me just understanding my pain and suffering. I never told her I wanted to die, but she has witnessed in her young years the hell that I have been going thru.
At that moment, I knew that it was not okay for me to give up! It is not okay to be selfish and take my life! No, I will not traumatize my kids and have that be their lasting memory of me. What I would leave them is a lesson that when you are at your worse, you take your life! That was not okay.

I decided that no matter what it takes, thru all the pain and suffering, that I will show my children you never give up, you fight!

What I realized at that moment was, I need to get my butt out of bed and find a cure or a solution to this autoimmune disease Psoriatic Arthritis and Psoriasis because the truth of the matter is, What if this awful disease hits any of my kids one day?

I need to know that my kids will not suffer like I did and that they will have safe options. It would kill me if my kids end up having this disease, so I will do my homework now to make sure there will be a safer alternative but most especially that they will always fight and have hope.

My Thoughts

I know that doctors out there are introduced to new drugs and we as patients are going to obviously try anything to achieve relief. Do doctors and pharmaceutical companies understand what we go thru or does it not matter? I know I sound like a broken record here, but it really makes you wonder. I think if we end up taking certain drugs and suffer side effects, our voices should be heard. You will hear me say this a few times in my book, but I am thankful to Eli Lily for inviting me to their forum to share MY story and to hear other stories from others who suffer from the same disease.

I was able to hear their similar story and how they to, wanted to end their life. For those who maybe reading this and having the same thoughts, have hope and fight! Don't sell yourself short and keep searching, don't give up because I guarantee there will be something out there to help you! It's hard, but keep positive! Most especially, find a support system that will lift you!

We didn't realize the extent of Illina's illness until she showed us photos prior to her treatment. We always admired her resiliency and positive outlook in life despite the ups and downs of her illness.
-Roy and Marie Powers

8 "EVERY TIME I GO INTO THE POOL, ALL THE KIDS WOULD LEAVE"

Being consumed with years of health issues, I have been trying to figure out why I have this disease, how did I get this disease, what am I going to do if my children ever get this disease? I never really thought about how Psoriatic Arthritis and Psoriasis does not discriminate against race or age or color just like cancer or other diseases out there.

I was at the Mayo Clinic for my month of natural tar treatment, The Goeckerman Treatment, when one of the nurses who tended to the patients that get light treatments told me about a young boy who was there for treatment as well. She said he was very quite and reserved. She spoke to his mom and told her about me and how I was a positive and upbeat person and asked her if it would be okay if I spoke to her son. She than came back to me and asked me if I would be interested to meet this young boy.

I was so excited and thought "Would I? I would be honored!" and just then I was thinking about how I never thought about kids having Psoriasis or Psoriatic Arthritis and how I just could not imagine them going thru this disease at such a young age.

It is unfortunate that Psoriasis is on the skin and visible. Kids can be mean, but come to find out from his mom, parents can be just as mean.

You would think that adults would be empathetic towards a child suffering with this disease, but if you don't have any knowledge about it, of course you want to protect your own child just incase the child with a body covered with sores was contagious.

If people don't know, we need to inform them and let them know that WE are not contagious and it is okay.
We need to EDUCATE.

When my new little friend agreed to meet with me, the nurse brought him over to my room and you could tell he was very nervous. We both had our hospital gowns on and I introduced myself and told him that I had the same exact thing that he had! He was the cutest thing, about 11 years old with big blue eyes. As I tried to show him my leg with my Psoriasis patches, I can tell he was trying not to look, but wanted to look and without turning his head his eyes caught a glimpse of my leg. I did most of the talking since he was very shy. I asked him if he has ever met anyone with Psoriasis and he nodded his head, No.

As I shared a personal story of how hard it is to go in public and how a family member was scared to hug me thinking they would get it, that definitely struck a cord because tears started rolling down his cheeks. I was like, oh no, are you ok? Has this happened to you?

He then shared how he would go to the community pool and as soon as he would go in, kids would see him and parents would tell their kids to get out of the pool! That made my heart break. I was so sad for him. Kids especially at that age could be so cruel.

What I told him was to try and not be sad or mad at the kids and parents who act the way they do because they don't understand and it was ok to let them know we are NOT contagious! I let him know that being positive was the key and to concentrate on what makes him happy. He told me he loved to draw and he loved the Minnesota Vikings football team. Now that made my heart happy and gave me an idea! I gave him a great big hug and walked him back to his room and then I met his mom.

I now understood why the nurses wanted me to meet with him alone. Talk about Debbie Downer! I left there in shock! Poor kid, no wonder he's depressed!

The Goeckerman Treatment is a great treatment offered at the Mayo Clinic. I love and swear by it and this would be my treatment of choice. It has been around for many years and it is a natural alternative to taking medication. The process is lengthy and could be covered by insurance but what may not be covered is housing or food for the month of treatment. I had researched what was a more natural alternative and found the Mayo Clinic to be the fit for me. They only offer the Goeckerman treatment in a few facilities here in the United States and the funding for this is small but needed especially for patients like us who are either to young or cannot tolerate drugs that cause side effects.

I was really fortunate to be able to get my month of treatment due in part of my husbands job called Cox Cares that was a relief fund for employees in need during difficult times. I know that it may have been difficult for my husband to ask for the extra help but at times you just have to put aside your pride especially when an opportunity comes along that you don't want to pass up. Cox Cares was a true blessing and we cannot thank them enough. I encourage anyone who may have to get a treatment that may seem out of reach financially to do your research and investigate every avenue especially thru your employers.

Back to Debbie Downer mom. When I met her she seemed to be a very nice lady. She told me the story of her son and his Psoriasis or let me rephrase that, She told me the BURDENS of her son to their family and continued to talk about her two beautiful daughters who were in dance class and how expensive that was and how having to come to Mayo Clinic for treatment for their son was taking away from the family! I was trying to change the subject and kept saying how great and positive this is for him because as she kept on wanting to go on, my little buddy was putting his head down feeling so bad. I can only imagine how many times a day she mentions that to him.

I was thinking, as a mother does she not feel for his pain? You can certainly see it physically on his skin. I then tried to tell her to just take a positive approach and if during their month stay here in Minnesota if they had ventured to all the beautiful spots right close to the hospital like the nature center or the fun parks and water ski shows all which are free!

I don't want to focus on the mom's negativity because I am sure it can be really hard on the whole family having to deal with his disease. I think it is just very important not to make him feel like such a burden.

It was definitely hard leaving the room. I just wanted to take him with me. This disease can put you in such a depression and for kids to go thru this is so heart wrenching. I decided to go to Walmart straight after treatment and make my buddy a basket of all his favorite things, since he would be there for a month. I had a couple of my girlfriends with me to help me find him a drawing art pad and some colored pencils, some fun Vikings memorabilia and some treats! We put the basket together and it looked awesome and I could not wait to surprise him the next day!

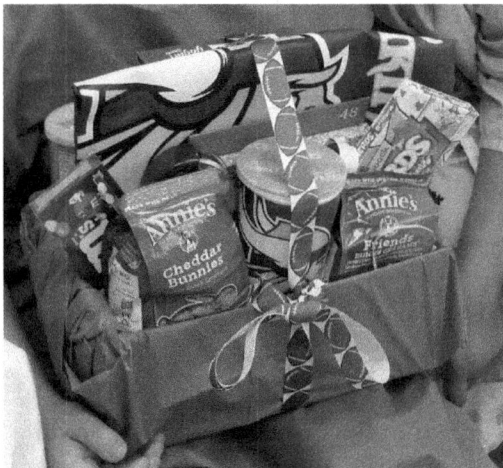

After giving him his basket, my nurse told me that ever since I talked to him the day before, that he was a totally different kid. She mentioned that no one had been able to get any kind of response ever since he started his treatment and how his mom was just so negative and how happy they were that he was able to meet someone just like him.

If I could live in Rochester Minnesota, I would love to be able to be a support guide to other patients especially young kids. This disease is tough and depressing and we just need to let people know who are not aware about this disease that it is ok to be around us and we are not contagious!

Sometimes you want to get mad but how can we be so upset if people do not understand. It is something we have to live with, but it is okay to have a voice and to educate. If we don't do it, then who will?

In todays age, if we are curious and want to learn about something we do not know about, we search for the info on the internet, and that too, is okay.

Always be mindful and think of others feelings. One of my quotes to live by is "Treat people the way you yourself would like to be treated". If you want people to be kind to you or treat you with respect, it goes both ways and does not matter if you are a young kid or a big kid!

My Thoughts:

It is so hard to go thru Psoriasis and Psoriatic Arthritis as an adult that I cannot even imagine going thru this disease as a child. Kids can be mean, but most especially if they don't know what another kid may have. As adults, we should not teach our kids to be afraid or stay away. It is okay to ask and as the parents of a child with this disease, do not get offended, and educate. Even us as sufferers should not be offended by people's comments if someone may ask us what is wrong with us. It is better that they ask instead of grabbing their child and running away. Yes, our feelings will get hurt but it will be one more person who will be educated. As a loved one to someone who has this disease, do not express all day what a burden it is to have to deal with them. We already feel bad. Stress is a big trigger for inflammation. It is very stressful to suffer from this disease. Especially, do not tell your child how time consuming and expensive or what a burden they are on the family. Look to be positive and seek out resources or support groups that may help the family out. The best thing you can do for a person going thru any disease not just Psoriasis or Psoriatic Arthritis is to be supportive. It makes a huge difference in a persons life suffering from any disease.

I am hoping that I made a little impact on my little buddy's life and that his one month stay at the Mayo Clinic will be memorable and that after seeing someone like him, he will not feel so alone. I hope the days at the pool when everyone runs away from him, he will not put his head down in sadness but lift his head and know it is okay to educate.

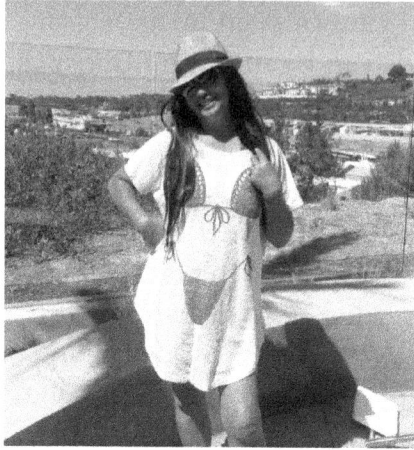

It is really hard to go to a public pool or to the beach in a bathing suit without people looking and wondering what is on your skin and if it is contagious. I try to find the positive and make light of my situation. It is what it is and I do not want psoriasis to stop me from enjoying life so I find other ways to enjoy pool and beach days. You will not ever catch in a bikini but you will catch me in my bikini shirt!

"Her will to survive is only matched by her will to be kind and giving to others" love ya sister...☐

-Dru Obrien

9 "WILL I END UP HAVING YOUR DISEASE?"

Hearing this question "Will I end up having your disease" is definitely disturbing. It is always my biggest worry as a mom who suffers from Psoriasis and Psoriatic Arthritis that my children can get this disease.

Is Psoriasis hereditary? It s said to be linked to genetics and having the gene doesn't mean that you will for sure develop the same condition but it may increase your risk for sure.

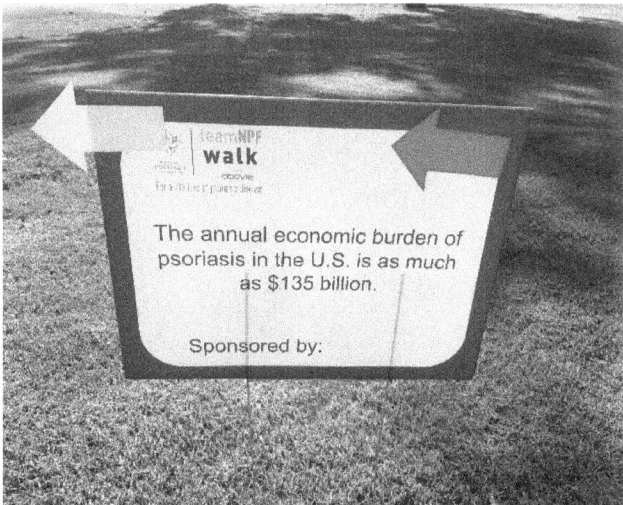

It is crazy to think, but about 7.5 million people in the United States have Psoriasis, Psoriatic Arthritis or both. If you have a family member like a parent who has this disease, there is a 10% chance of getting it. If both parents have it 50% chance of getting it.

Drugs for this disease is not for everyone and the drugs I took that I may have got a side effect from may not affect other people in the same way. Our bodies are all different and we react to things differently.

If I knew there was something out there that would be safe for treating this disease, I can rest easy. This has been a journey filled with side effects that it scares me to even think that my kids can possibly wake up one day and have Psoriasis, Psoriatic Arthritis or both! I do not want them to suffer like I did.

To have my kids watch me suffer for so many years just makes me so sad. We were talking one day and the kids were reminiscing about what they remember growing up and it seems that their memories have been of me being around, but not really. I was not able to do regular mom things because I was in pain and the kids had to grow up fast and do a lot of things for themselves. I understand why there would be a fear. I feel awful and see the stress especially in my daughter's eyes.

If there is something not in the norm, I see her questioning it. Why is my skin dry? What is this mark? Is it Psoriasis? My son says his knees hurt, Do I have arthritis? I try to reassure them, but you can't help but wonder.

When my kids are around, I do find myself doing a check from their head to their toes to see if I see patches or anything that may indicate signs of Psoriasis. At times I would ask myself, "How did I hit the jackpot and get both? It really sucks and I just don't know which is worse? The excruciating pain from the arthritis and not being able to walk or dress myself or write or start the car? Or is it the embarrassing sores that cover my body that itches and feels raw, bleeds and everyone stares. But I don't have to pick which is worse and hope that I had one over the other because I have both! Sometimes I can't even differentiate what pain is it that I am feeling. Its hard to explain but sometimes I feel multiple pains at one time. My toes are swollen the size of sausages along with the bottom of my feet and I cannot walk. My knees hurt, my fingers are huge and also the size of sausages! My joints are red and hot while my wrist are stiff along with my spine and my neck!!!! I am telling you, the pain is like no other and I am surprised I just do not pass out. There is no Tylenol, No Advil no pain killer that even help.

In fact, it adds other symptoms and makes me feel worse that I pray to be admitted to the hospital or just pray that I don't wake up. I never want my kids to feel this pain.

I remember one day going to a family party and and one of my nieces hesitated to give me a hug asking me if she were to touch me, would she become like me and get my disease. I was surprised and shocked that she would think that, but I had to remind myself that she is young and does not understand. My daughter who was maybe 6 at the time immediately said "I hug my mommy all the time and I don't have what she has."

I was curious why she would think that so I asked her, "Who told you that?" and she said her mom, which would be my sister.

I was even more confused, and a bit hurt and I was anxious to join the party. I was hurt because I had no idea why my sister would tell her daughter that. What people do not understand and maybe thinking is, Oh my gosh, she is being so sensitive and dramatic, but for a person who all of a sudden acquires this disease, you already feel so embarrassed, ugly and self conscious.
People stare and for those who are not educated about this disease, you have to remember to educate before getting upset.

It is a natural reaction if people look at you and think you maybe contagious when that is not the case at all. I found myself covering up from head to toe and after awhile, I felt it was best just to stay home and not join the family parties. I felt that if my own family did not understand, then it was better for me to just stay home.

I was not at the point where I was able to share out in the open that I was NOT contagious since this was even new for me. Sometimes I was starting to miss family events and they did not understand and I would start hearing things like, Is she really sick or if I was pretending to be sick. When you see me I looked normal since I was covered up, but what was I to do? Strip my clothes for them to believe me?

I really started to pull back and regress. I just wanted to be in a corner because my skin was all over the place and I can see and feel how people would stare. It was getting to the point where people were thinking what a snob I was and how I was being anti-social, but when really I just did not know how to deal with a life of Psoriasis and the severe pain of the Psoriatic Arthritis. I could see that I was slowly losing my friends and family. Those who could not understand and would judge. It was a very hard time for me. Some times I would attempt going to a party but I would look in the mirror and watch the skin from my head drop all over my clothes and see the sores bleeding on my head or even blood coming thru my clothing. How was I to feel going out in public? But I would try to put a brave face and pretend I was okay when really, I was screaming inside. This is something that I knew scared my kids and I would die if they ever had to go thru what I have gone thru. I remember how people would start to pick the huge flake out of my hair not knowing it was the flakes from Psoriasis. They were so big, it did look like something fell or flew into my hair and someone would say "Oh, stand still, you have something in your hair."

I would get so embarrassed and go to the nearest restroom and just cry. Even though I have been going thru this for so many years I especially felt so sad when my husband looked at me. I am not the girl he married years ago and now he gets to deal with this.
I would not blame him if he were to find a new partner in life who is healthy and can walk and looks beautiful. This is just something that pains me and I wish that some day soon there will be something for me so I can live life with my husband.

When I shared my story with a little boy from the Mayo Clinic who was getting the same Tar Treatment as I was, I told him that someone asked me if they were to touch me, would they become like me, tears started to roll down his face. I knew that struck a cord and that he could relate. Kids are kids, they are honest and truthful, but I'd like to think as an adult, especially a family member, they would make an effort and do a little research before sharing or scaring others that they may get my disease from touching me.

I get it, It's scary, I do look contagious, but don't stay away. It is my mission to have a plan incase my kids may one day wake up and realize that they too have Psoriasis or Psoriatic Arthritis to find safe and healthy options on treating this disease and to be aware of drugs that always have side effects. I cannot say DO NOT take these drugs because until you have suffered this horrible disease and there is no other option but to take these drugs in order to have some quality of life. I can only guide them and teach them how to eat the right foods to keep them healthy and take their vitamins and keep active because I do believe after years of seeing what works and what doesn't work, Diet makes a big difference. Staying away from processed food and sugary foods and inflammatory foods makes a big difference. Keeping on an Anti-inflammatory diet will only help to not trigger Auto-Immune diseases to come alive!

I also encourage my kids to live life every day and do fun stuff because you just never know when it will hit you. One day I am okay, and next day I am in a wheelchair. We should never wait until something bad or traumatic happens before living life. Keeping positive especially during the hardest times is the key.

Instead of worrying "Will I End Up Having Your Disease?" Live Life and enjoy friends and family!

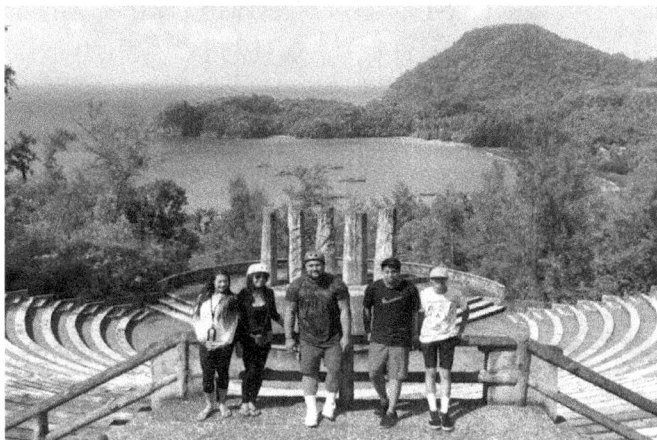

10 "AFTER INSURANCE AND COPAY, YOUR PRESCRIPTION WILL BE $3000"

Excuse me, I'm not sure if I heard you correctly? Did you mean $300? This was the latest exchange of conversation I had with the Pharmacist at my local pharmacy when I went to pick up a newly prescribed medication by my Rheumatologist.

I find it very entertaining that when I walk into the pharmacy they know me by name and greet me with a "Hi Illana!" I told them that I wasn't sure if it was a good thing that we were on a first name basis, But for as much as I am there, how can they not know my name. I'm not going to

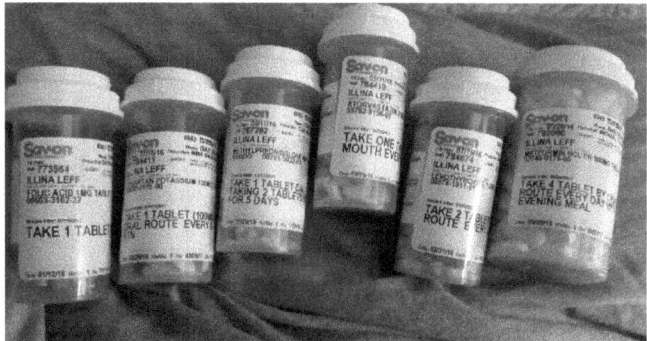

lie, It's a good feeling to know that they know ME!

This isn't something new and has been going on for years now. How is it possible that Pharmaceutical companies can charge what they do to us patients who need these drugs? I have had to deal with this issue one to many times and have had to deal with this for years. The struggle I have been thru in order to get approved or to be able to afford some of the medication prescribed to me has been such a battle. I would always think to myself, "If I am going thru this, I know there are millions of other people here in the United States going thru this as well!" What do they do? How can they afford it?" For myself, I would go back to my doctor and let them know how much they are charging me and that I cannot afford to pick it up. The sad thing is, I do have a great insurance plan and with my co-pay it still cost me an arm and a leg! If I am lucky, my doctors may have samples to get me thru until I get approved months down the line.

I remember years back when I was going thru my chemo therapy for my Non-Hodgkin's Lymphoma and I was very nauseated from my chemo, so my Oncologist wrote me a prescription for an Anti-nausea medication. It seems easy enough, so I made my way to the pharmacy to pick it up, so I thought, until I was told that it would cost me $900! Basically if I did not want to violently throw up and feel nauseated after my chemo treatments, I would need to pay $900! What's wrong with this picture? I can NOT afford that, so what was I to do? I literally told my family, forget that, I'll just suffer! I was on other medications as well that cost me about $150 a month and that alone was a struggle. I knew at that moment I was feeling very sick and I needed something that would help calm my nerves and stop the nausea and vomiting.

The girl at the pharmacy suggested that maybe I buy a few to get me thru the week and that was over $100. It is so mind boggling how these pharmaceutical companies price out their drug. At times I feel like doctors also just prescribe one drug after another so they can get some kind of kick back. I started to understand how this whole thing worked after I found out that the Doctors at Mayo Clinic do not get these same kick backs and maybe that is why they are not shoving down prescriptions down your throat. I guess you can say I am angry, who wouldn't be.

There were also a couple times when I was prescribed a biologic to help my Psoriasis and Psoriatic Arthritis but was told it would be over $500. I would be given a coupon and after bringing it to the pharmacy, I would be told that they did not accept it and to contact the pharmaceutical company directly. My doctor's office would also try to fill out paper work to see if I qualify to receive it at next to nothing. Sometimes it would take months to even get an answer back while I continue to suffer.

At one time I was hopeful because I did qualify to receive a package of my biologic injections delivered to my home. Things seem to be going well and I was nearing the end of my 12th injection so I thought I should renew my prescription. Come to find out, the coupon was good for a discount for the first 12 injections. The only way to continue taking these injections would be to pay $500 and that is with my insurance and co-pay. Let me clarify, it would cost me $500 an injection that I needed to take once a week for the rest of my life.

Is that how that works? You take this drug that changes the quality of your life, I can walk again, my skin has cleared up all the sores and you find this miracle drug that has changed your life. It is like a teaser, you take it and you just know that you do not want to go back to the pain and suffering. The pharmaceutical companies know that they can hike up the price because you won't be able to live without it! Is that fair? Not really, will they continue to do that? I have been going thru this over 10 years and seems like nothing has changed. I hope to make it to Washington D.C. one day to have my voice heard, not just for me but for others who suffer from this dreadful disease. It is just not fair.

It's okay, I did not need to continue taking the injection since I started to have a terrible cough that was getting worse every day and I ended up being diagnosed with Cancer...Non-Hodgkin's Lymphoma. Which I mentioned in another chapter as what a coincidence. I cannot prove if the reason I got Lymphoma was from this biologic, but like I said, what a coincidence since one of the side effects stated on their commercial or on the product says "May cause Lymphoma".

I tried to stay away from taking any new prescriptions that was being prescribed to me because I'm not going to sugar coat it, I was scared of what will happen next! Eventually my Rheumatologist persuaded me that there was something new unlike the previous biologics that I have taken.
He told me it is safer and no need for blood test and the worse that might happen would be mild stomach aches even though thru my research it also said to let your doctor know if you have suicidal thoughts or depression.

I was already depressed from everything! Would that mean I would get more depressed then I already am and all the suicidal thoughts that come thru my head may be a reality from this new drug? Oh my gosh! It may not happen but remember, I have been deemed the Poster Child for Side Effects! Of course I think that will happen to me.

Once again I am desperate, my skin is all over the place, anywhere I sit or sleep there is just a trail of skin. I want my husband to touch me again, to feel my soft skin and maybe just maybe if I try this new drug which again my doctor said it is safe. This may just be the magic drug! He gave me samples for the month, so I will give it a try while his medical assistant makes calls to the pharmaceutical company once again to try and get me approved on receiving this hopefully at no cost. Until that comes thru though My doctor called in a prescription to my local pharmacy.

Of course I am very hesitant and I stare at the samples for a few days. I have to psych myself out and give myself a pep talk in order to take this new drug. I am hopeful and I say a prayer that it will work and to please, please, please let there be no side effects. Also, Since the warning label is included I'll go ahead and read it to make sure I am aware what to look out for. This is the name of the game, this will forever be my life, and it is horrible what this can do to your mind.

So here I am greeted at my local pharmacy "Hi Ilana!" They never get my name right but they are so sweet I just say Hello back. "Hi Ladies! I have a new prescription to pick up along with other prescriptions if they are ready please!" I could sense something was wrong by the look on her face. How can I explain it? It was a look of shock and laughter at the same time as the sweet Pharmacist says to me "After your insurance and your co-pay it will cost you $3000" and that is when I said

"Excuse me, I'm not sure if I heard you correctly? Did you mean $300?" and she verified that I heard correctly the first time, it was $3000!

Here I am again, I started the samples, I'm not seeing any significant changes since I just started taking it but I do get stomach cramps but it just does not matter. $3000??? Are you kidding me? Even if it were $300 I still could not afford that!

My thought every time this happens:

If a drug like this is $3000 and a doctor prescribes this and you get it filled, how much does he get? Just curious. For the pharmaceutical companies out there, what goes behind the price of medication? Just curious. Could it be because this is not a drug needed for life or death purposes and it is for cosmetic purposes even a person with Psoriasis or Psoriatic Arthritis suffers in pain from their condition.

Just when I thought it could not get any worse from $500 to $900 to $3000!
I know that doctors are just doing their job, diagnosing their patients and they have to pretty much trust the pharmaceutical reps who go to their office and give them information why the doctors should SELL or I mean prescribe THEIR super drug. I guess they can only go by what they are told or what they read about that drug and the clinical trial studies.

Sure, that drug might be a miracle drug for other sufferers, but at one point do they step back and add up all the side effects, the cancers or the deaths? Is it still considered safe? And when you call the pharmaceutical directly to express your sadness or anger about what happened to you, they just pass you on to a customer service rep who takes a report and you then become a statistic. Or you get the doctors who want to cover themselves and tell you that the cancer or heart failure that you encountered can't possibly be related. Really?

I am angry, I do want my voice to be heard. It is not ok, what are in these biologics that you even have to say on the warning label "May cause Lymphoma" and I coincidently get Lymphoma but it's not from the drug I am told. But here I am fighting for my life.

I especially get a kick from when I enter different Walks like the Arthritis Walk or Psoriasis Walk or Cancer Walk and I go up to the booths that manufactured Enbrel or Humira or Stelara and share with them my experience and they just stare at me with a blank stare and say "Oh, I'm sorry, I have not heard that." You mean to say that I am the first person to tell you that I was told by my doctors that I was in the last stages of Aids, or Got Lymphoma or

Heart failure right after I tried a Biologic? You mean as a Pharmaceutical rep your company has not shared the stories of the patients who have suffered an adverse side effect?

Well, if the companies do not want to hear my voice after leaving messages, then you bet I am going to give these reps a lesson so they can be aware. If they are shocked to hear what I have to say, I am shock they they have nothing to say or pretend they have no idea what I am talking about. Educate your reps! I hope once you read what a real person goes thru after taking your over priced drugs, you will have a little bit of compassion instead of thinking of the prize, the pay day.

Again, my book was made possible from the opportunity Eli Lily gave me as an invited guest to speak in their forum and share Our story. They really took the time to listen to people with Psoriatic Arthritis and Psoriasis and our pain and suffering so they will understand when they market their Drug. What they did was so powerful and I suggest these other companies follow suit. For Eli Lily I am so grateful, Thank- you for hearing our voices when others choose not to.

"Shocked and amazed at what Illina has prevailed through. You are an inspiration to us all."
-Jennifer Baker Kozicki

11 BLESSED BY ANGELS

Angels come in all shapes and forms and you can be a believer or not, but in my life time I have been a witness to a few moments that I believe I was blessed by an Angel.

My Angels came to me in the form of my friends who really got me thru some pretty tough times and I will never forget their act of kindness that would lift my spirits and take me out of my place of darkness.

I want to share a few stories because if there are others in the same situation who may not realize Angels around them, this may shed some light.

When I was first diagnosed with my cancer, Non-Hodgkin's Lymphoma, I remember my sweet neighbors who pulled together and brought us meals to lessen the burden when I started my chemo treatments. That was such a blessing and you just feel the love and support that surrounds you. I had a dear neighbor named Darie who has always been so bubbly and funny and just a positive energy who came by with a check and told me that she did not know what our family likes to eat, so if maybe my husband can take her check and go to Costco and pick our favorite meals. I was so touched and thankful. However, my husband had a look on his face of horror and I thought

"Oh my gosh, how rude!" He could not understand what was going on. You see, this was the first time that either of us at our young age had been hit with cancer. It was a shocker to us and to everyone around us. I was in my 30's and I had a toddler along with 3 other kids under the age of 11!

We were not familiar with the process of Cancer and what happens, but apparently, people come together to show their support. My husband on the other hand, thought I may have gone thru the neighborhood with a collection basket announcing my cancer. After having a conversation with him, I was able to understand that my husband's feelings were hurt and his pride was bruised by our neighbors bringing checks, money and food. His first impression was that people thought he would not be able to take care of his family. The truth of the matter was, he had a great job! We just never experienced something like this in our young lives and it was so humbling to get the support we did. It meant so much.

I also had one of my girlfriends who lived about an hour away and just dropped everything, like she always does for me and took charge of my home and my family and I liked it! All of a sudden, my sister from another mister, Silvia and her family blessed my home with love and she had a selection of wigs for me AND whipped up dinner and left overs and dessert to last us for the week! It was little things like this that made me feel that every thing was going to be ok. I also remembered when I came to the end of my chemo treatments, I sat in my same chair hooked up to my I.V. in a room filled with other patients receiving their chemo treatments when she showed up with a bouquet of balloons to celebrate my life and getting thru my months of chemo! Even to this day, when I accomplish something like getting a new job, she sends me a bouquet of flowers or fruit! She is a positive light in my life and truly and angel!

What my close circle of friends did not realize, was there were days I felt so alone and afraid. I would get to that low point where I could not walk, could not care for my family and I did not want to burden my family anymore but I also did not want to be that Debbie Downer that every time a friend calls me I would cry and they would have to hear my pity party and feel helpless. I just felt so bad. I remember looking at myself in the mirror, my skin filled with sores from my Psoriasis, my body was filled with horrific pain and I could not even move. My husband would have to carry me to the bathroom or the kids would hold me up to sip out of a straw, I just did not want to live anymore. How can I put my family thru this? I felt I had a reason to justify why I should take my life! This was not a quality of life!

I remember looking around and the vacuum was next to my bed so I can easily vacuum up my skin, but there was one day I thought, maybe I will just tightly take the cord and wrap it around my neck so I will stop breathing or maybe I will take the pain meds and sleeping pills and just not wake up. At those moments I would all of a sudden get a call from a friend I have not heard from in awhile saying they are checking up on me. It seemed to be my friends Sabrina and Kathy A that would have an intuition and call me at he moments I had these thoughts. It was odd, but I felt my angels needed to transport thru them to get me back on track. I would cry and they would listen and give me the hope and strength I needed to get thru my day. I had this feeling that my guardian angels would work miracles thru my friends. I then decided to do something really crazy and I made a video of myself, as a diary log. I felt so compelled to share it with a few friends. I was at my worse and I was very emotional and I knew I did not want to commit a selfish act and have my kids deal with their mom taking her life. I just could not do that to them! What will that teach them? I want them to see that no matter what, I will fight to the end. If there was any message I could share with my kids or anyone out there who is in despair, As bad as it may seem, taking your life is permanent solution to a temporary problem. **Please Seek Help**.

So back to this video I sent out. Maybe these close friends were wondering, Why in the world would she share this personal and raw and disturbing video? My dear friends, I felt so alone and I wanted to get out of this dark place and I knew I had these awesome girlfriends who would lift me from this darkness. How would they know that I wanted to take my life because of my suffering unless I shared it with them. I was not looking for pity sending this video out and I am truly sorry if I made you all feel uncomfortable, but I sent it because I would do more to cover up and pretend I was not sick or that I was okay and they did not really know how bad I was. It was so important that I had my close circle of friends understand and give me the strength to fight thru this and not feel so alone. I am lucky to have my friends always come thru for me and I feel like that is a big reason why I am here today sharing my story.

I want people to know that when you have a loved one going thru something so traumatic, it may be easier if it is out of sight, out of mind or maybe you are scared and feel helpless, but trust me, that hand you may offer might just be that life vest that helps save a life, in this case it was mine.

Other then that, just having the core friends that talk to you on a daily basis to see how you are saves your soul everyday. The little get together we have make me realize how blessed I am.

This next Angel hit me from no where. You will like this story. It was about half way thru my chemo treatments and it had been a hard beginning of the year. We had just lost our business, and about two weeks after, I was diagnosed with the "C" word CANCER, Non-Hodgkin's Lymphoma. It was a financially tough time for us and it came at a time when my oldest son Noah, was preparing to go on his Washington D.C. trip in 8th grade. Then one day I got a call from the tour company saying that final payment was due for Noah's Washington trip and I totally forgot! I mean I was a little busy going thru my chemo treatments. I decided that I would take on an a job waitressing at a local 24 hour diner so I can collect some good tips to help pay for his trip. After losing our business, I just did not want to burden my husband with another thing. My Oncologist found out that I started a new job and advised me that might not be a good idea since my immune system was low and I was still going thru chemo treatments.

He said I needed to get stronger and healthier. I explained to him that we just lost our business and that I needed to do this for my son and my doctor completely understood and gave me the okay.

The following day, I followed up with the tour company to see if they can just give me a week or two to come up with the rest of the payment when they said "Ma'am' I believe you are all paid up", Your son is good to go and there had been an over payment. Should we mail it back to you? I thought, finally my ex-husband made a payment and I told them to go ahead and send it back to him. The lady then said, "The name does not match" I was very confused. I then asked them what was the name, and they said FONG. I literally fell of my chair in tears! I was like Fong as in my Dr. Fong? I told the lady on the phone my story how I was going thru chemo right now and that Dr. Fong is my Oncologist and she started to cry with me! The next day I went to my sons school and spoke to Mr. Jerome, the teacher in charge of the trip and asked him if my doctor came and spoke to him and he denied it but I could tell he was not telling me something until I said, I knew what he did because I spoke to the tour company and that is when he said "Yes, ok, Your doctor came here to the school to drop off a check and told me not to tell you." My Oncologist Dr. Fong, went to my sons school and paid off my sons trip to Washington D.C.!

You heard right! What doctor does that? I was in complete disbelief and brought to tears and every time I share that story, like on the airplane to strangers we part and they are crying. An Angel? Absolutely in my book.

Even though I can go on and on with how I have been blessed by and Angel, I feel like when a person goes thru some challenges in their lives, it no longer ends up being a gloom and doom life and sometimes these blessings come to you because of what you are going thru or have overcome.

Another day I felt such a powerful positive energy surrounding me that I remembered posting on Facebook that I should buy a lotto ticket or go to the casino because for some odd reason I was feeling really lucky. All of a sudden I received two phone calls and an email which brought me good news! All in the same day. The email stated the I was hired for a job with the airlines, the first phone call was that I was chosen to be part of a speaker's forum to share my story about my journey for having Psoriasis and Psoriatic Arthritis and the next phone call was that I was chosen to be on a documentary about someone who was an Energy Healer and he would like to help me with my pain and other issues on his show.

I think I may have texted all my friends letting them know how odd that day was but I was going to embrace it!

Being a guest for Eli Lily Pharmaceutical Company opened my eyes to life as a Psoriasis and Psoriatic Sufferer. They helped me to open up and share my story which is why you are reading this book today. The pain of trying to remember everything I have gone thru caused me 9 years of writers block. After I shared my story in a room filled with other people who had my same disease, they told me that my story was very compelling and that I should write my book. They validated that my story was worthy, in fact everyone there that day who shared their story was worthy.

It was surprising because I have tried for years to be heard by the other pharmaceutical companies which I coincidentally suffered a side effect from and not one person would take the time to listen to my story and I believe I was just another statistic in their reports. I want Eli Lily to know that even though I have never taken any of their drugs, what they do partnering up with the National Psoriasis Foundation and inviting people who suffer from Psoriasis and Psoriatic Arthritis to share their story is such an awesome and life changing gesture.

Last but not least, this next experience has changed my life and I am still on cloud nine! Ever since I was diagnosed with Psoriatic Arthritis I have experienced a pain like no other. Some days worse than others, some days I would be using a walker and wheelchair and some days I am able to walk. But for any given time, I am always in some kind of pain. It sucks! I feel like I have tried everything from Tylenol to pain killers which cause me to suffer a side effect to different Biologics. My feet, knees, toes, elbows, wrist, spine and fingers are always inflamed.

When I saw an ad online, They were looking for people who suffered from chronic illnesses and pain. I immediately thought "Hey That's me!" There was a brief description that a new show was going be filmed about a young guy who was an Energy Healer and was looking for people who fit the profile to be in his show for a chance to help with pain. Of course I was curious but also a skeptic. I have never heard of an Energy Healer. I have seen shows in the past where a healer may put their hands on you at church and then all of a sudden they would pass out. Was it going to be like that? I thought, what can I lose?

I have tried so many different drugs which I coincidently suffered a side effect from, what can go wrong?

I filled out the questionnaire and the next morning I was asked to come to the Burbank/Hollywood Studios for an interview and a few weeks later I was chosen by Charlie, The Healer, to receive a healing from him.

The day of filming there must have been about a crew of ten setting up in my home. We were nervous and anxious to meet Charlie. When he finally arrived, he was straight and to the point and asked me where my pain was and I went down the list. My toes were like sausages, ankles are in pain, elbow felt like fire, both wrist felt like I had carpal tunnel and my spine was throbbing. He looked at my fingers and said to me "It looks like you already have joint damage, I'm not sure if I will be able to help you but we will give it a try.

As he held my arm, his eyes started to flutter and I suddenly felt a warmth that took over my body. I always tell people that is felt like taking a balloon and rubbing it on your hair and your hair sticks straight up, like static. I was nervous and I wanted it to work, but I was also nervous if it didn't work. All I knew was that I was not about to pretend on national television for 8 million viewers to see! He then told me to walk around and tell him how I felt. In my mind I was thinking, Is he serious? It has taken almost 9 years to try and come up with the right treatment. There is just no way that he would just flutter his eyes and then like Magic, I'm healed!

I did what he told me and I got up from the couch and walked around. I wiggled my ankles and they were not cracking nor could I feel pain. I just kept on saying how weird this was. I did not know how to react because I was still skeptical about this so called, Energy Healing. My body felt good, but I was scared to say it felt good because was it going to last for a few minutes and go away? I was really weirded out! I had so many questions but I was being filmed and then I all of a sudden I shrieked and told everyone to look at my swollen joint damage fingers! In fifteen minutes the inflammation was going away and it was visible proof. I don't understand what was going on but I was so happy it just did not matter! Everyday I waited to see if the pain would come back. Six months later I am still feeling good! One year later still no inflammation in my joints! The Psoriasis on my skin was still there but not having the pain on my joints was heaven! I just love Charlie Goldsmith, my own personal Healer…My Angel!

I think this is my longest chapter and I can go on and on and mention everyone who has touched my life like the doctors, interns and especially my nurses who cared for me at the Mayo Clinic everyday for a month, I just love them so much because it truly takes a special person to become a nurse. They were so kind and supportive and baked my family cookies and got me a beautiful bracelet before I left. Every time I looked at each of them they had halos above their heads! Mayo Clinic Rochester is my happy place and I hope to find a home there one day.

I can go on about my girlfriends Keri, Dru, Rachelle, Sheri and Kathy who always came to my rescue when I could not walk and literally carried me or helped me with my kids. Or Amy, Linda, Lynnann, Kristy, Sabrina, Quin, Roy, Marie, Jennifer, Genelle, Kira, Laura or Susan who always had an ear or shoulder for me to cry on.

My neighbors thru the years who became my family I cherish your unending support.

Or Catherine and Jackie who accompanied me to Mayo and saw me at my worse whose support meant so much. I know we say we love our friends, It's important we have our friends, but to me these are my Angels and I have been truly blessed…Blessed by Angels.

12 I'M THANKFUL FOR MY STRUGGLE BECAUSE WITHOUT IT I WOULDN'T HAVE STUMBLED ACROSS MY STRENGTH

I think that we can all say that we have struggled in some form, wether it may be struggling on a homework assignment, struggling financially, struggling in a relationship or in my case, struggling with health issues. The strength comes by how you perceive and handle the obstacles that come your way. It is pretty much a given to say that an average person will go thru some kind of stressful situation in their life time, some more than others, but how we deal with that struggle is the key.

Some days I would just cry and say how horrible my life is and lay in bed under my covers and justify my thoughts of taking my life and how I would do it. Another day I would knock some sense into my crazy thoughts and tell myself "C'mon, this is not you, this is not what you want your kids to know you for." Do I really want my kids to know that because of my pain and suffering, there is only one option and that would be to take my life? NO!!! I want them to know that even thru the toughest time we fight and never give up! I am so glad that I did not believe that my ugly skin and arthritis pain was my only destiny. I did not say "Well I have Cancer so I give up, I am going to die." What I am trying to say is, take every single ounce of energy you have, no matter how much it will drain you and come up with a positive plan.

It does not have to be a grand plan, but make it a positive plan. You will be surprised of your true strength.

I always thought to myself that I could not continue living like this and having my husband and kids carry me to the bathroom or get me dressed. This cannot be my life and there has got to be something out there to change this. I went back to my doctors and told them to please, try to fix me AGAIN! I was not going to accept that this was my fate. Most importantly, Do not take this on all alone. Let your friends or family know you can use some support. That is an important key factor to take you out of that dark place, especially if you are having negative thoughts taking you places you should not be going. What ever you believe in, you need to believe. For me it was prayer for strength to get me thru.

Never ever give up and feel like you have to accept that there is only one plan if that is what your doctors are saying, especially if it is not working for you. My Rheumatologist at one point seemed to get his ego hurt when I told him that I was going to search for a place that specialized in Psoriasis and Psoriatic Arthritis. I found myself having to explain how I have followed their plan for 7 years and I am getting worse and it was hard when they would tell me that I am the worse case patient they have or that I am top worse in the nation. I just wanted to go to a place where they have seen other patients like me.

I live in California but I found a way to get the second or third opinion that I needed when I went to Oregon and NYU in New York and finally The Mayo Clinic in Rochester Minnesota which really saved me.

I wasn't sure at the time how I was going to make it to these places since our funds were limited, but once again I had an angel whose little ears were obviously listening at my doctors appointments and it was my then 9 year old son who came to me when I was in the hospital for two weeks and said "Mom, I made you something". I assumed that maybe he made me a card, but he handed me his phone. It was a Gofundme that said "Please Help My Mommy." I was filled with emotion and thinking bless his little heart. He has had to watch me suffer for so long. He said he wanted to start this Gofundme so I can find a doctor that can help me since I was the worse in the nation. Right there I knew, his little ears were listening during my appointments. In one week he raised $1000 and in two weeks it reached almost $5000! Needless to say, I was able to find a doctor and a plan that helped me.

Your life is worth it, I am so glad I did not give up. I am in a whole different place and I am able to share my story and hopefully give hope.

Nine years ago, I can remember saying "I need to write a book" and started the process of writing this book. But every time I would put the pen to the paper, I struggled. My emotions would always get the best of me. I thought that the biggest struggle in my life journey was from my auto-immune disease Psoriasis and Psoriatic Arthritis, or from different side effects like Cancer Non-Hodgkins

Lymphoma or heart failure, or the yearning to have the support of family. However, It seems that my biggest struggle right now would be to figure out how was I to share all the years of pain and suffering, the memories of coming close to death and bringing awareness and educating Doctor's and Pharmaceutical companies of the reality of what a person that suffers a side effect goes thru after taking a drug that has been prescribed.

When I had the pleasure to meet others who suffered from an auto immune disease at an advisory board that I was invited to by a well know pharmaceutical company Eli Lily, I noticed that the one thing we all had in common was how each of us had a story to tell and our voice needed to be heard and not ignored and Eli Lily gave us that platform to share.

What happened that weekend, I would have to say, changed my life and it was what I needed to start healing. Being at this forum allowed me to hear stories from people also suffering and it was eerie to hear the similarities. It was hard to hear that they too, in their darkest days, also wanted to "Jump off that bridge". I was not sure until that day, if my story was worthy or compelling enough, but I did know, that if I can be that one voice that will give one person hope during their time of struggle, My heart would be full.

Suffering from a debilitating disease for years bottles up every kind of emotion from being mad, feeling sad, having a pity party, happy when things are good and our body suffers. Not everyone may want to write a book about their journey but maybe writing in a journal will help to heal and release the pain. My goal is to have mini forums where we can get together and share our stories. It is a good thing to meet others who have walked in your shoes, they understand exactly what you are going thru.

Find a local support group and share. You will be amazed how much strength and healing that will bring you.

The struggle it would take to look at myself in the mirror, would always make me cry. I looked ugly and felt ugly. Again I would take everything I had to keep positive and I would moisturize my dry skin from my psoriasis and then go thru my closet and pick something out that would be comfortable but cute. Just because I had Psoriasis does not mean I could not look cute. This is where people could not understand and would say to me, "I never knew, you always looked okay." Obviously, I don't go around flashing people my skin! This is what I meant by how we handle our stresses. Taking a little time to feel good or look good or smell good will do wonders for your self esteem during an already stressful time.

With my arthritis as bad as it was, the pain was excruciating and debilitating. When my kids would have to help me get dressed I couldn't help but cry. This is not supposed to be happening, I am only in my 30's. I could not even start my car and the kids were late to school and at times I could not even get them there. I really, really tried my hardest though, to do what I had to, even if it took me 30 minutes to walk from my bedroom to the car. There were times I found myself calling my friends in desperation for help. I did not want to burden anyone but I had to swallow my pride and ask for help. Having strength can be picking up the phone and swallowing your pride. It is very hard to make that decision. You don't want to bother anyone or have the fear of asking and they might say no.

Always know that you are stronger than you think. When you are thinking "I can't, I Can't!" turn it around and say "I can, I can!"

It has been 10 years of Struggling from Psoriasis and Psoriatic Arthritis and everything that comes with it but I make sure to remember and count my blessings. It is tucked away in my mind but I make sure to revisit each and every memory of my struggles, not to relive that pain and suffering but to celebrate that I fought thru each one and is the reason why I am here today able to share my story.

After I made it thru my chemo and I was finally in remission, I realized that God has given me my life to live and that I am very blessed. I want to heal and live my life, be happy and give back. Going thru a life threatening illness puts life in a whole new light. The material things did not matter as much anymore.I knew what would make my heart full and it was doing for others.

I decided to volunteer at my local Make-a-Wish Foundation and I am going on almost ten years now volunteering to help kids with life threatening illnesses get their most heartfelt wishes. I became a wish granter and a speaker for them. I was not ready for what was in store for me, but it was good. Being able to meet each and every family and each special wish child was exactly what saved me. I knew that my life with my health issues was tough, but when I realized what these families were going thru, it put things in perspective and I could relate and understood that being here today gave my life purpose. My family also became very involved, my husband became my wish partner and my kids started a Make-a-Wish Club at their school.

The biggest struggle which I know I spoke about in one of my chapters was not having the support from family. Not my immediate family kids and husband, but my siblings. For years I could never understand it. I really thought that as family that is what you do. Going thru my cancer and chemo and not knowing wether I would make it to the next day, I had hoped I would have got their support to especially help me with my kids.

That was such a hard time for me and for whatever reason they could not be there I have learned to forgive them for my inner peace. I learned to build a support system with the friends around me who understood and wanted to be there for my family. That meant the world to me.

One of my favorite quotes by Alex Elle

I'M THANKFUL FOR MY STRUGGLE, BECAUSE WITHOUT IT I WOULDN'T HAVE STUMBLED ACROSS MY STRENGTH!

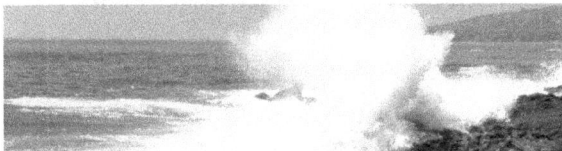

I am very thankful.

ABOUT THE AUTHOR

ILLINA LEFF is a two-time Cancer Survivor and has battled Psoriasis and Psoriatic Arthritis going on eleven years now. She lives in the beautiful beach town of San Clemente and is a wife to her Junior High School Sweetheart Bob and a proud mother of four kids to Noah, Josh, Ryann and Nate. She loves her dog Gigi, a Standard Poodle and rescue Kitty, Bindi. She is passionate about helping others and has been a Wish Granter and Speaker for Make-a-Wish Foundation going on ten years now to help kids going thru a life threatening illnesses. As a sufferer of an Auto-Immune disease, Psoriasis and Psoriatic arthritis, ILLINA has made it her mission to bring awareness to this disease and to let others who are also suffering know that 'You are not alone!" She loves to travel and hopes that someday soon she will be able to tour and share her story and have a forum for others to also share their stories.
"Life is unpredictable and we just need to live it!"

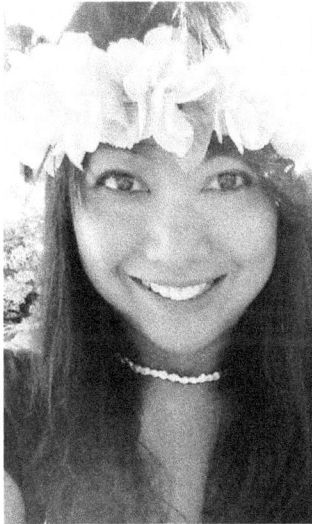

Contact thru Instagram #illinaleff_Stillstanding
Or Facebook IllinaLeff_StillStanding@PsoriasisandPsoriaticArthritis

www.ingramcontent.com/pod-product-compliance
Lightning Source LLC
Chambersburg PA
CBHW071138280326

41935CB00010B/1275